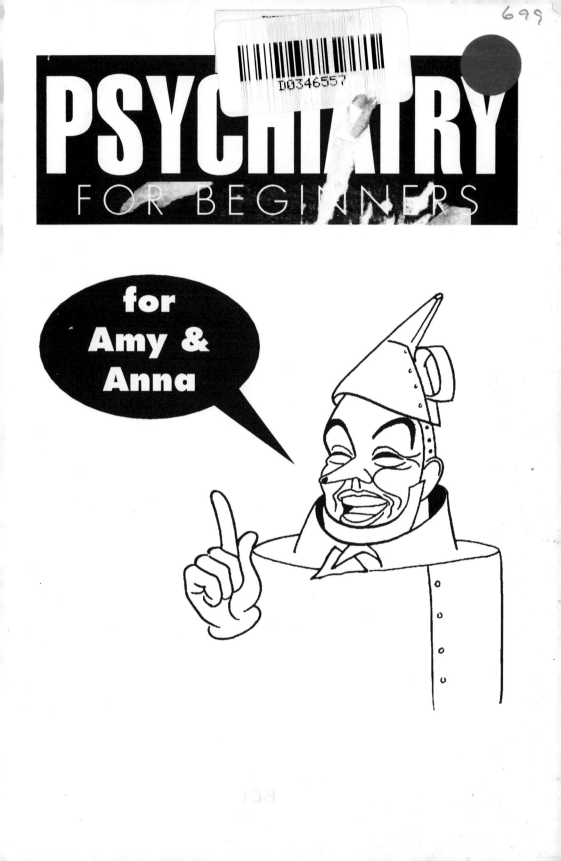

699

WRITERS AND READERS PUBLISHING, INCORPORATED

P.O. Box 461, Village Station
New York, NY 10014

c/o Airlift Book Company
26 Eden Grove
London N7 8EF
England

A Writers and Readers Documentary Comic Book
Copyright © 1993
Library of Congress Catalog Card Number 93-60875
ISBN # 0-86316-166-9 Trade
1 2 3 4 5 6 7 8 9 0

Manufactured in the United States of America

Beginners Documentary Comic Books are published by Writers and Readers Publishing, Inc. Its trademark, consisting of the words "For Beginners, Writers and Readers Documentary Comic Books" and the Writers and Readers logo, is registered in the U. S. Patent and Trademark Office and in other countries.

PSYCHIATRY

FOR BEGINNERS

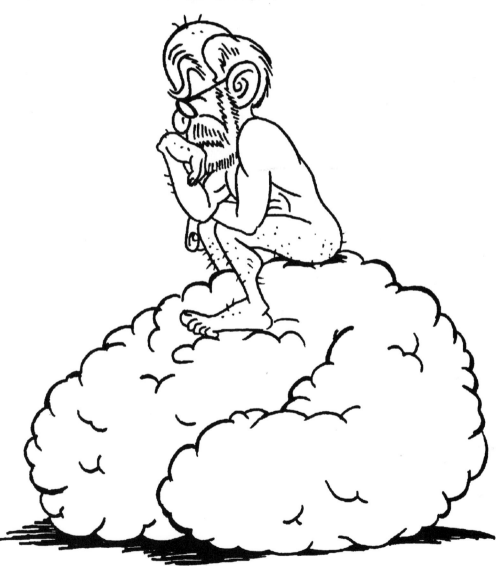

FROM TIME IMMEMORIAL...

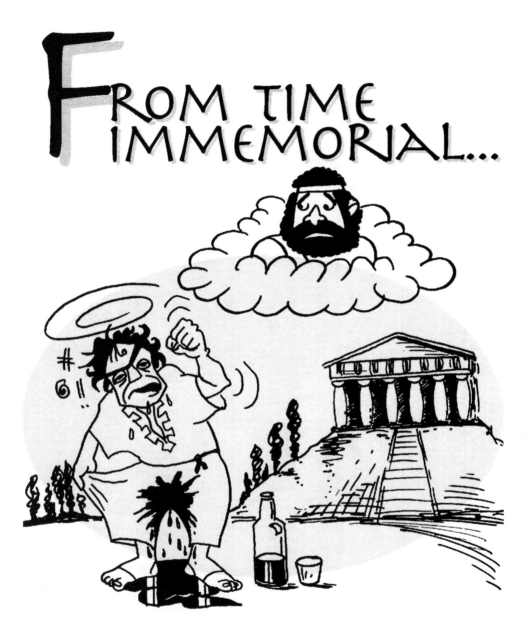

...men and women have been prey to confusion.

•

The ancients blamed many of their troubles on the
Gods, who could be either vengeful or rewarding,
depending on the deities' whims.

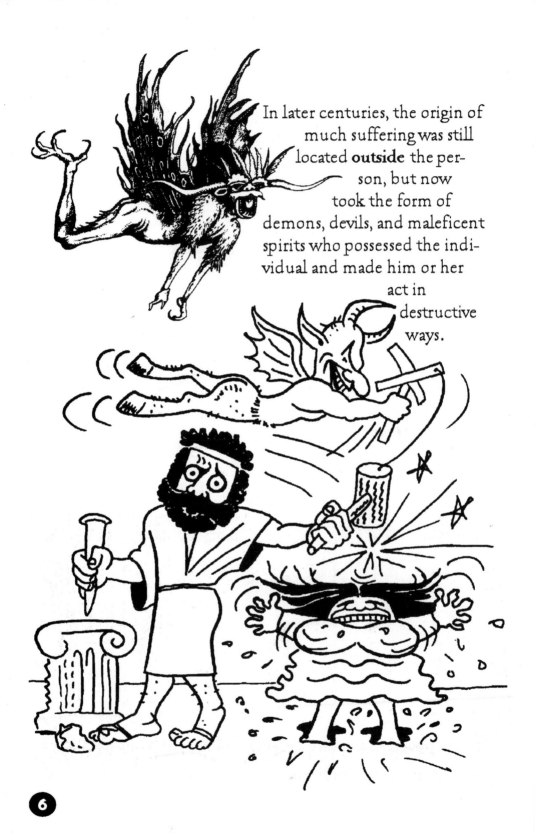

In later centuries, the origin of much suffering was still located **outside** the person, but now took the form of demons, devils, and maleficent spirits who possessed the individual and made him or her act in destructive ways.

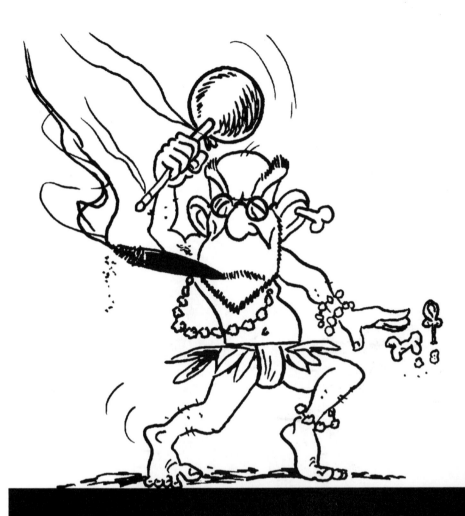

Eventually though, explanations of good and evil, of cause and effect, became increasingly ANTHROPOCENTRIC. Men and women were seen not only as the object but also as the source of a good deal of their suffering.

With an internal—that is to say, human—origin of pain, the shaman, the medicine man, the exorcist, became irrelevant. Unnecessary. A new type of healer, a healer of the inner world, of the PSYCHE (Greek: the soul), came into being: a secular priest known as a PSYCHIATRIST.

With some exceptions, the psychiatric approach relies heavily on the individual. The individual is seen as both the source and the potential healer of his or her problems. 'Patients' come to 'doctors'—psychiatrists—not only with problems like anxiety, guilt, and depression, but with homelessness, poverty, joblessness and other social ills. The psychiatrist, who has been trained to fit his observations into a 'medical model', attempts to diagnose and treat such problems, regardless of their ultimate (political or social or economic) origin.

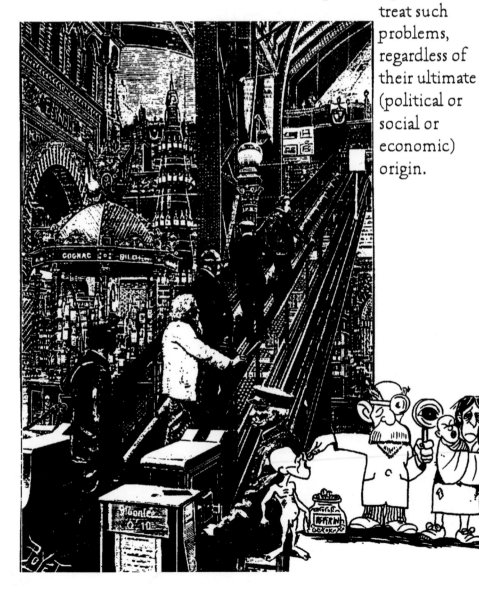

This lets government off the hook. Those who for one reason or another remain disaffiliated, peripheral, unable to fit into the mainstream as productive members of society, can be viewed as 'sick', as victims of disease who require medication or even institutionalization.

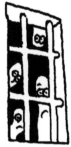

STATE HOSPITAL

GRIND I MUST

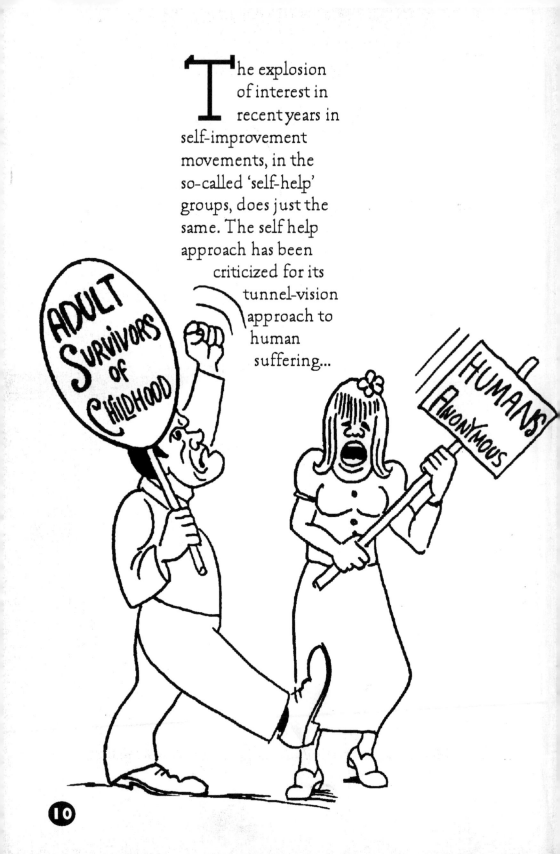

The explosion of interest in recent years in self-improvement movements, in the so-called 'self-help' groups, does just the same. The self help approach has been criticized for its tunnel-vision approach to human suffering...

So what exactly IS psychiatry?

"the branch of medicine concerned with the study and treatment of disorders of the mind, including psychoses and neuroses."

-Noah Webster

the handiwork of the devil!

-Joseph Smith, Mormon

a capitalist ploy, created by and for the bourgeoisie, to keep the focus off of class struggle.

-Karl Marx

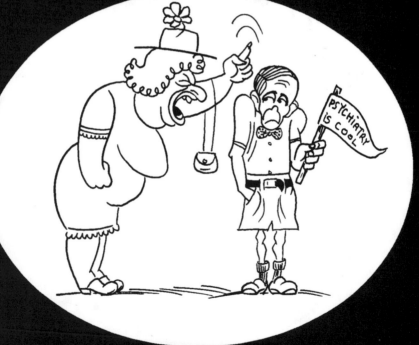

"You lie on a couch and you don't even face the person and for this you pay money? it's nuts, crazy i tell you, who needs it?"

-My Grandma Rose

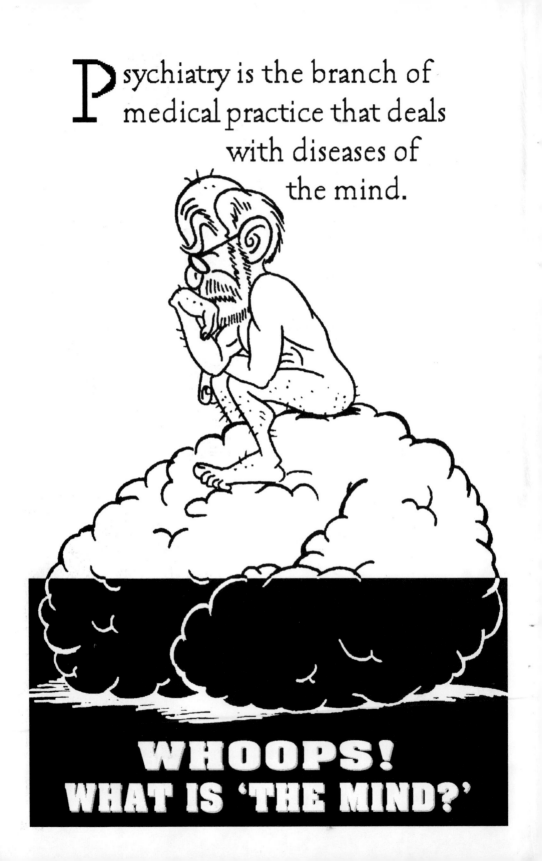

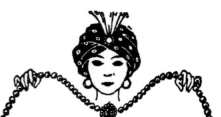

Right—forget that. Philosophers and psychologists and religious thinkers have been trying to answer that one for a long long time. And still haven't succeeded. Let's try again:

Psychiatry is a medical specialty that deals with disorders of the brain.

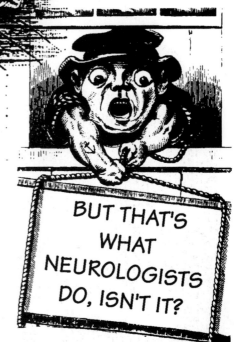

BUT THAT'S WHAT NEUROLOGISTS DO, ISN'T IT?

Psychiatry is the medical specialty that diagnoses and treats disorders of mood, thinking, and behavior.

BUT THAT'S WHAT PSYCHOLOGISTS & PSYCHOTHERAPISTS DO! WHAT'S SO SPECIAL ABOUT PSYCHIATRY?

Unlike the psychologist (whose doctorate [Ph.D.] in psychology earns him the title of 'Doctor'), or the psychotherapist (who can be a social worker or nurse or other type of counselor), the psychiatrist is a physician (medical doctor, M.D.) whose professional training includes four years of medical school plus additional years in psychiatry. Unlike other mental health practitioners, psychiatrists are trained to recognize physical illnesses which can cause or contribute to emotional ones.

Psychiatrists can prescribe medication for their patients. Psychiatrists tend to ask a lot of questions. The mental health 'consumer' owes it to him or herself to be well informed, and should be prepared to ask some questions too.

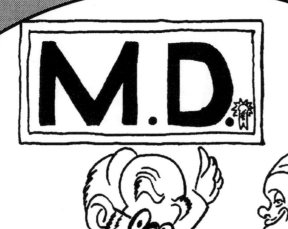

L

et's turn the tables. Let's visit a psychiatrist and ask some questions of our own.

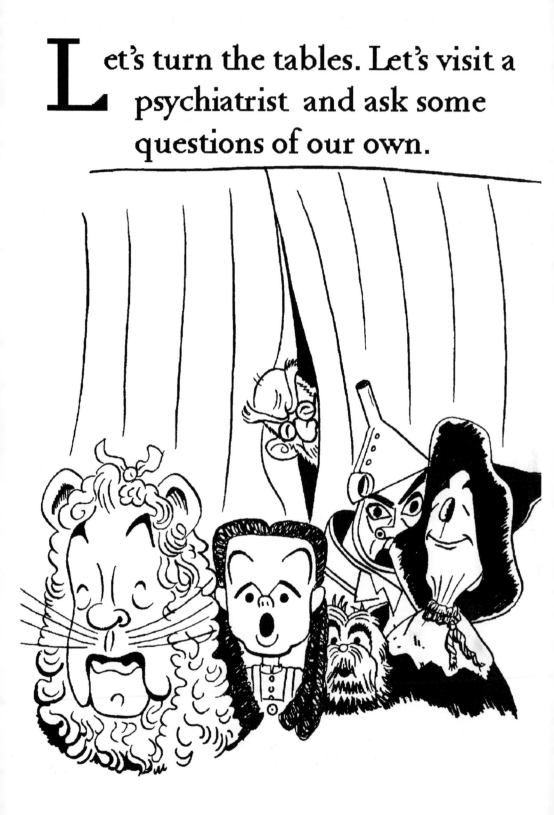

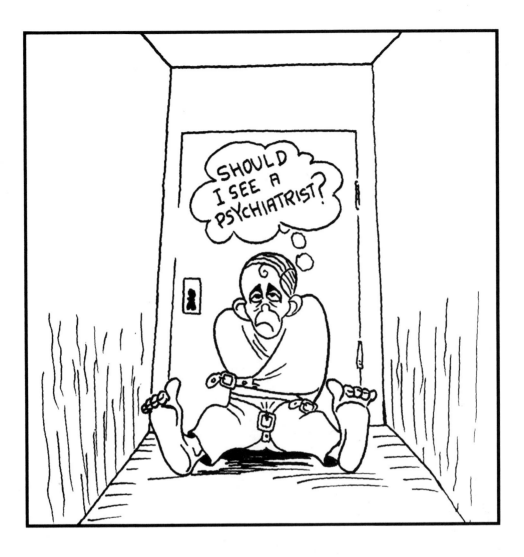

How did it all come about? Did psychiatry always exist?
What are psychiatrists like?

Why are they called *shrinks*?

What do they do?

Do psychiatrists in Bora-Bora practice
the same as ones in Brooklyn?

Should I see one? And if so, when?

And how will I know which one is right for me?

The popular notion of the psychiatrist—as a pipe-smoking tweed-jacketed observer, given over to infrequent and often ambiguous commentary—is a relatively recent one.

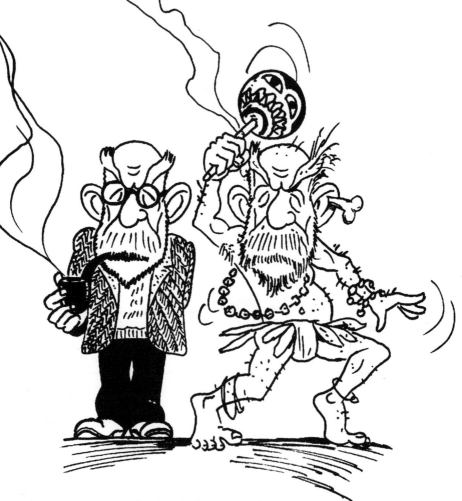

Primitive peoples had their psychiatries too. Through various means, including deliberately induced trance states and suggestion, prehistoric medicine men (**shamans**) practiced hypnotism and acted as **mediums** to bring about supernatural interventions on behalf of the sick.

The Old Testament records that Saul had recurrent severe depressions. Ezekiel was coprophagic (ate fecies.) David escaped from captivity by pretending to be mad.

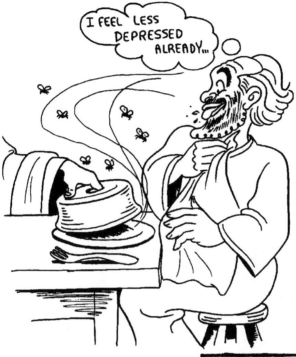

The scriptural association of madness with evil (Leviticus: "...*a man also or a woman that hath a familiar spirit, or that is a wizard, shall surely be put to death...*) has been used to justify the torture and murder of the mentally ill throughout history.

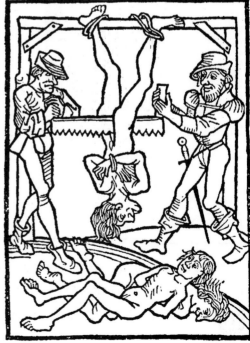

The Hindu writings of ancient India abound in references to mental phenomena and problems. According to Susruta, passions and intense emotions could cause both mental and physical diseases. The individual personality reflected the preponderance or relative lack of the four 'primary' elements, fire, water, earth, and ether (air.) Mental problems were referred to the priest. Sound familiar? It is only later, with the Greeks, that we begin to see attempts at a rational or scientific approach to mental illness.

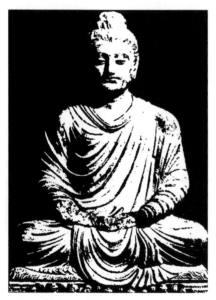

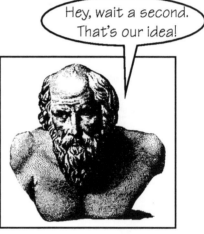

Hey, wait a second. That's our idea!

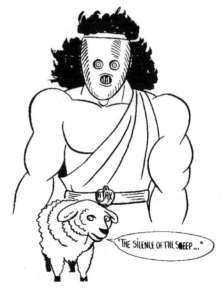

"THE SILENCE OF THE SHEEP..."

Greek mythology is chock full of tales of madness and mental woe: mental illness as punishment by the gods...Ajax, in a fit of madness, slaughtered a flock of sheep; Orestes hallucinated furies, which only he could see.

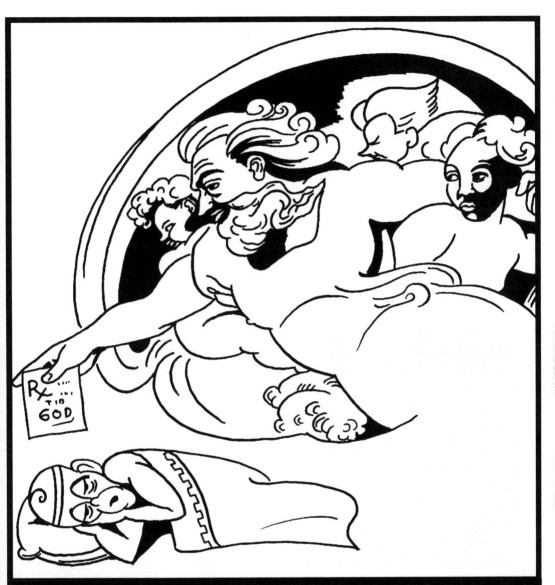

The mentally infirm among the Greeks were treated with ORACULAR HEALING. The patient would sleep near the Aesculapian temple, and be visited by—that is, dream—of the god producing a cure.

•

Visions and hallucinations were occasionally seen as divine; this early association of unusual mental phenomena and religion laid the groundwork for the widespread hatred and fear of the mentally ill.

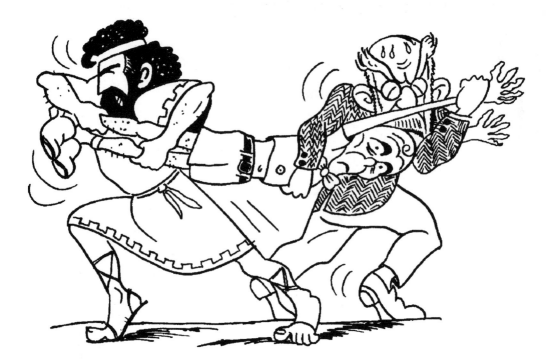

The Big Picture: in ancient Greece, the mind and its problems were the exclusive province of the philosopher and priest. Until **Hippocrates** came along and stated that such problems were strictly medical.

Hippocrates on epilepsy (which in those days was known as the 'Sacred Disease'): *"It thus appears to me to be in no way more divine, nor more sacred than other diseases,"* and *"They who first referred this disease to the gods appear to me to have been just such persons as the conjurors, purificators, mountebanks and charlatans now are...such persons...use the divinity as a pretext and a screen for their own inability to afford any assistance."*

Hippocrates compiled what are probably the earliest written descriptions of the symptoms of depression, and offered a coherent classification of mental diseases, including mania, melancholic depression, paranoia, and hysteria.

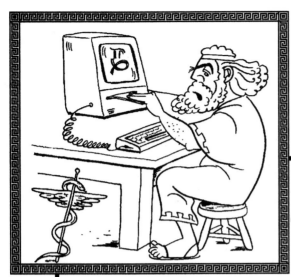

One more mental disease and I'll have to expand the memory!

Hippocrates' anatomic (as opposed to theologic) view of mental problems was not entirely progressive, however. He still subscribed to the theory of **humors** (body juices.) Personality in both health and disease depended on the exact proportion of black bile, yellow bile, blood, and phlegm in the individual's makeup (sound familiar?) The brain's normal functioning depended on a harmony between the humors. An excess of bile could lead to anxiety, or melancholia. Predominance of one or another of the humors led to distinct personality types, or temperaments: the *phlegmatic, choleric, melancholic, and sanguine…*

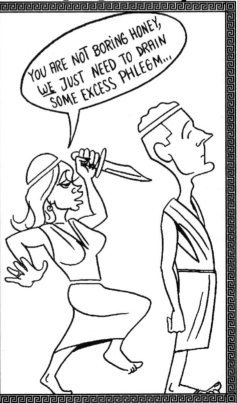

YOU ARE NOT BORING HONEY, WE JUST NEED TO DRAIN SOME EXCESS PHLEGM…

Breath (**pneuma**) was viewed as the ultimate source of intelligence and feeling, although it was with the brain that we thought, dreamt, and felt.

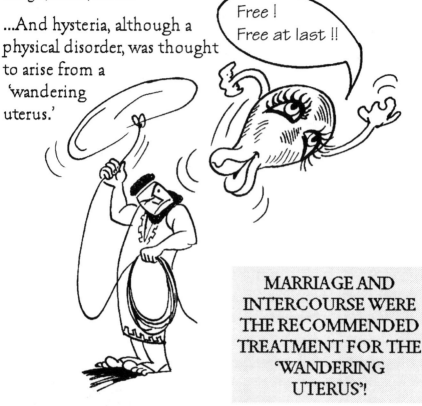

...And hysteria, although a physical disorder, was thought to arise from a 'wandering uterus.'

Free!
Free at last !!

MARRIAGE AND INTERCOURSE WERE THE RECOMMENDED TREATMENT FOR THE 'WANDERING UTERUS'!

Unfortunately, Hippocrates' view of the brain's central role in mental illness and health was not championed by subsequent thinkers. Aristotle, Epicurus, and Zeno and others continued to look upon the heart as the origin of psychological activity.

Plato (427-347 B.C.) took a giant step backwards, insisting once again that madness could either be of divine origin—sacred—or merely ordinary. The rational part of the soul was in perennial conflict with the appetitive part. Mental suffering could be alleviated by a dialogue, or dialectic, between patient and physician.

24

Another inheritance from the early Greeks (the Stoics) was the idea of *tabula rasa*--that man is born as a clean slate, with his character 'written' over the course of time by his accumulated experience. This notion lies at the heart of the nature vs. nurture controversy, and is at odds with later views on the heritability of certain mental characteristics and disorders.

Aristotle (384-322 B.C.), a pupil of Plato, played a large role in 'physicalizing' mental illness. Psychological troubles had to have a physical basis. The brain's major function was to condense the hot vapors arising from the heart. (Giving rise to the idea, so popular in later centuries, that nervous problems were caused by 'vapors.')

EXCUSE ME...
MY HEART IS REALLY ACTING UP

Aristotle also claimed that all great thinkers had a 'melancholic temperament.'

Giving rise to yet another controversy, still unresolved today: are creative people more prone to depression, mood swings, and mental illness?

METHODISTS: abnormal contraction or expansion of body organs resulted in illness.

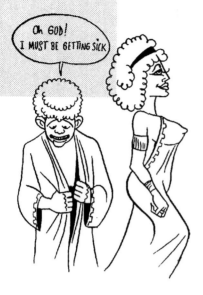

According to the Epicurians and Stoics, mental illness was the result of unsatisfied passion and desire.

Asclepiades. a Roman physician (first century B.C.), added to psychiatric knowledge by separating acute from chronic conditions. He also distinguished delirious states (due to fever) from mental conditions without accompanying physical illness. Asclepiades objected strongly to the then current practice of confining the mentally ill in cells and dungeons. Predating Esquirol (a French psychiatrist of the 19th century) by some twenty centuries, Asclepiades also differentiated between *delusions* and *hallucinations*.

> **Delusion: A firmly held belief not shared by most individuals in one's culture.**

i.e., 'Insanity is caused by demons' would not have been a delusion back in prehistoric or medieval times.

> **Hallucination: A visual or auditory perception which is unapparent to all except the person experiencing it.**

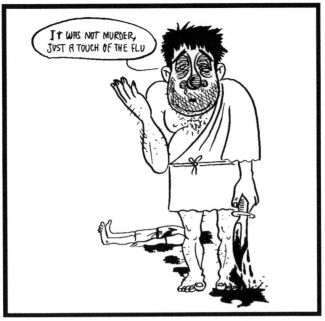

THE ROMANS

Cicero: suggested that criminal and other deviant behavior was due to 'sickness.'

Roman law established the precedent of legal incompetence for the mentally ill.

These ideas were echoed many centuries later by **Thomas Aquinas** (1225-1274), who reasoned that the soul, being divine, could not become ill; therefore insanity was a somatic (= physical) disorder, and the insane could not be accountable for their behavior.

Plutarch's description of the melancholic is just as relevant today:

> "...every little evil is magnified by the scaring spectres of his anxiety. 'Leave me', says the wretched man, 'me the impious, the accursed, hated of the gods, to suffer my punishment.' He sits out of doors, wrapped in sackcloth and filthy rags. Ever and anon he rolls himself, naked, in the dirt confessing about this and that sin...Nowhere can he find an escape from his imaginary terrors."

Cornelius Celsus, a Roman physician, insisted that mental illness involved the entire personality and not just one bodily organ. [*Yaaa!*] He also advocated the use of fetters, sudden fright, and bloodletting for treatment. [*Boo! Hiss!*]

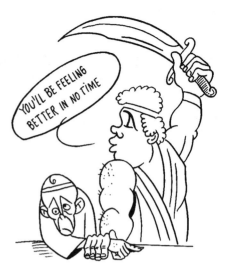

Around 50-100 A.D., physicians began to notice that mania (abnormal states of excitement) often preceded or went along with states of depression. Some, such as **Areteus of Cappodocia**, paid more and more attention to *prognosis*, the prediction of the outcome of illness.

Areteus of Cappodocia:

> "It is impossible, indeed, to make well all who are ill; for then would a physician be superior to a god."

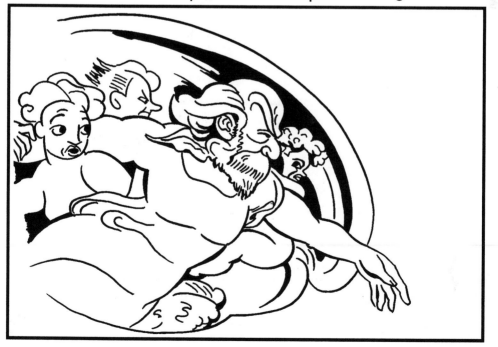

Certain disorders, such as mania, had a self-limited course, while others were chronic and untreatable.

<u>Soranus' description of a maniac:</u> "the patient may imagine he has taken another form than his own; one believes himself a sparrow, a cock, or an earthen vase; another, a god, orator or actor, carrying gravely a stalk of straw and imagining himself holding a sceptre of the world; some utter the cries of an infant and demand to be carried in arms, or they believe themselves a grain of mustard and tremble continually for fear of being eaten by a hen; some even refuse to urinate for fear of causing a new deluge."

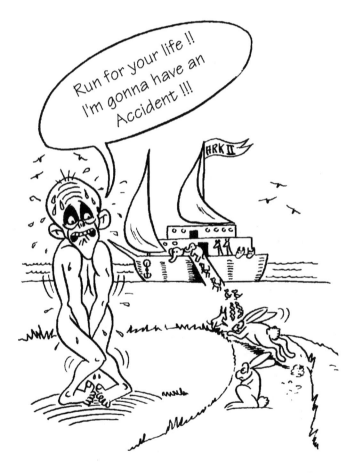

With **Galen** (130-200 B.C.) we see the rise of *eclecticism*, an attempt to combine traditional approaches with more contemporary developments.

GALEN'S CONTRIBUTIONS TO PSYCHIATRY INCLUDE:

His *positivist* (that is, based on strictly observable facts) approach: "Do not go to the gods to make inquiries and thus attempt by sooth-saying to discover the nature of the directing soul...or the principle of action of nerves; but go and take instruction on the subject from an anatomist."

His notion of affliction by consensus, or sympathy: symptoms in one part of the body may be due to disease in another part... psychological disorders could cause physical ones.

Among the earliest (animal) experiments demonstrating that the brain was the center of sensory and motor function.

Diseases were caused by negative influences from the environment such as poor nutrition or bad air.

Galen's Rx pad: blood letting, purging, diets, exercise, and the intentional contraction of 'quartary fever' (probably malaria).

"Those ancients were pretty clever. Seems like many of our 'modern' ideas about psychology date back to the Greeks and Romans."

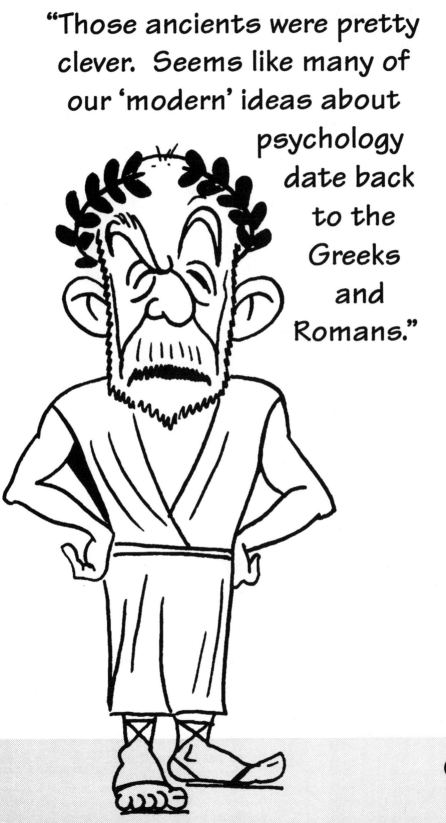

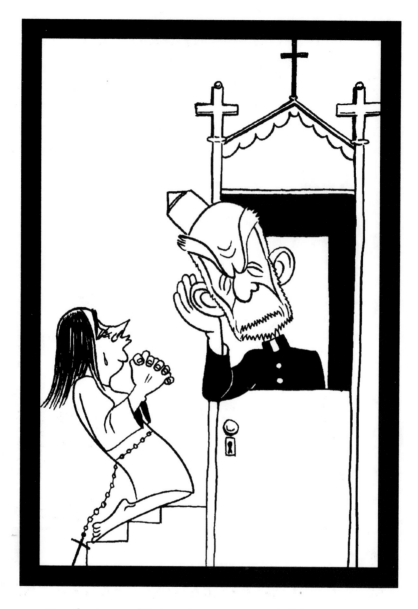

Confessions of Saint Augustine (345-430 A.D.):
featuring psychological self-disclosure;
forerunner of psychoanalysis?

Incidentally, the Greeks and Romans didn't have a
monopoly on psychiatric thought. **Avicenna** (980-
1037), a renowned Muslim physician, noted that
emotional factors could cause physical illness.

Original psychiatric thinking in Christian Western Europe during the centuries following Galen was sparse. Physicians relied either on the work of Hippocrates and Galen, or returned to earlier superstitious views. Humoral theories (and worse--such as theories of demonic possession, evil astrological influence) were once again invoked to explain illness. Available treatments were hardly better: folk medicines, specifics recommended centuries earlier by Hippocrates and Galen, even exorcism by priests...

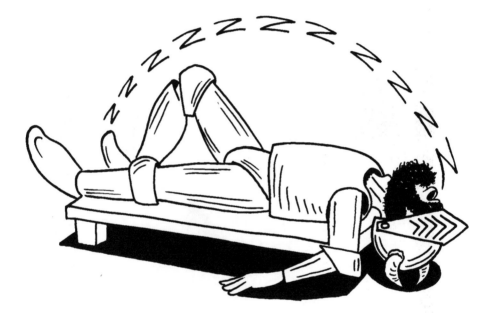

And how's this for eclectic:

Phillipus Aureolus Theophratus Bombastus von Hohenheim, otherwise known as **Paracelsus** (1493-1541), a widely celebrated physician and alchemist, wrote that mental illness had a natural cause...but he also recommended that the insane be burned (better the stake than the devil!)

As far as the mentally ill were concerned, the Renaissance was in many respects merely a 'Renaissance' of scapegoating and superstition. At the same time, however, the Renaissance saw a renewed and invigorated search for natural rather than supernatural causes of mental illness, with increased emphasis for example on the concept of *imaginatio* (=suggestion), a force able to both cause and cure mental illnesses.

WHERE THE REMEDY IS WORSE THAN THE DISEASE: The Pope's designated Inquisitors, Kramer and Sprenger, devised a manual, the *Malleus Maleficarum* (1486), for the 'diagnosis' and 'treatment' of witchcraft.

Thousands of so-called 'witches' (in reality, women who were either eccentric or delusional or hysterical or simply unlucky enough to be on the wrong end of the accusing finger) were burned at the stake for their 'crimes.'

"I've got just the thing for what ails you".

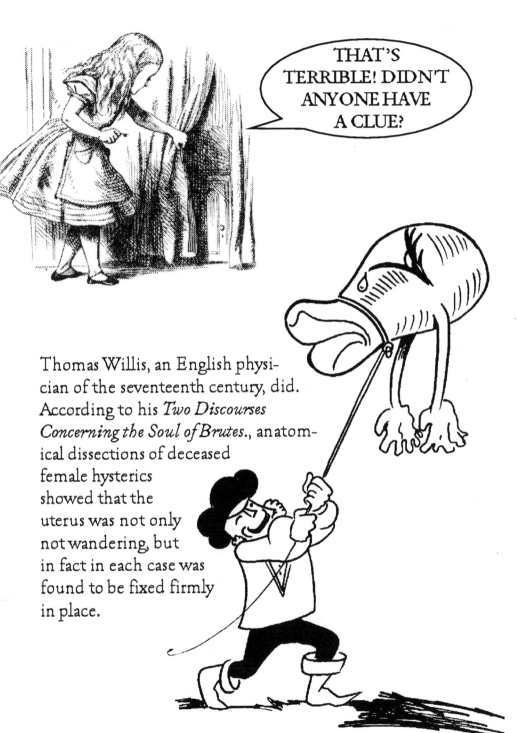

THAT'S TERRIBLE! DIDN'T ANYONE HAVE A CLUE?

Thomas Willis, an English physician of the seventeenth century, did. According to his *Two Discourses Concerning the Soul of Brutes.*, anatomical dissections of deceased female hysterics showed that the uterus was not only not wandering, but in fact in each case was found to be fixed firmly in place.

"Okay, already, enough with the stake and the torture and the exorcisms... How about *hospitals*? Were there any hospitals for the medieval insane?"

Muslim wards and hospitals for the mentally ill were established as far back as the eighth and ninth centuries. Psychiatric hospital care in Europe begins in the thirteenth century. The fifteenth century saw the rise of several Spanish asylums of note. The rise of these institutions is probably the most important development in psychiatry in medieval times.

The prevalent attitude during the eighteenth century was that mental illness was incurable. The insane were relegated to asylums, often for life, throughout Europe. An English Act of 1774 stipulated that the institutionalized should be... cured!

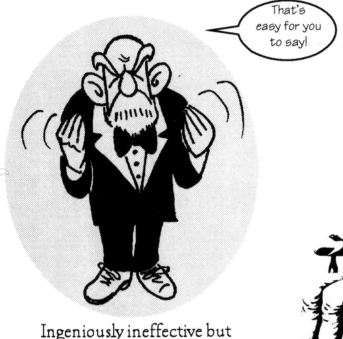

That's easy for you to say!

Ingeniously ineffective but cruel treatments continued to hold sway in these asylums, including dunking, starvation, bondage, and threats. For a few pence, the English citizen could actually witness the insane on display in the Bethlehem asylum.

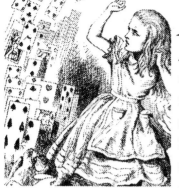

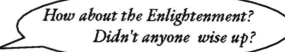

How about the Enlightenment?
Didn't anyone wise up?

Actually there were some promising developments. Doctors began classifying mental illness more systematically than ever before. **George Stahl** (1660-1734), a German physician, separated those diseases that had an organic (=physical, or bodily organ) basis from those that were functional (or as he would put it, 'of the soul.') **Morgagni's** autopsies on mentally ill patients helped further this development.

With the discovery of the nervous system, previous explanations based on 'vapors' or humors could be discarded and individuals could in good faith be said to be suffering from 'nerves'...

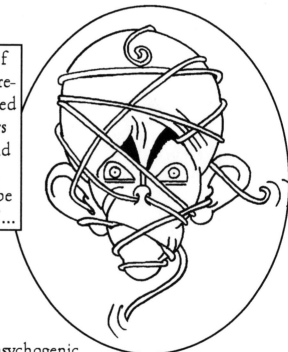

In the eighteenth century, sociological and psychogenic theories of mental illness arise.

Toward the close of the eighteenth century, **Phillipe Pinel** in Paris, Vincenzo Chiarugi in Florence, William Tuke in York, and Langermann in Bayreuth, spearheaded dramatic reforms in the asylums.

At the Bicetre and Salpetriere asylums, Pinel liberated the inmates from their chains and insisted on humanitarian (what he called 'moral') treatment of the insane.

Inspired by the French Revolution and its Declaration of the Rights of Man perhaps?...'

Tuke (1784-1857) championed his moral treatment of the insane, advocating strongly for nonrestraint of the mentally ill.

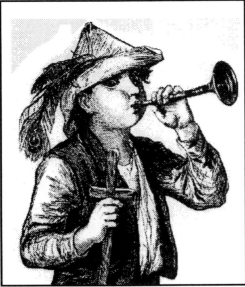

Pinel's approach really was revolutionary. His description and classification of mental disorders into mania, melancholy, idiocy and dementia was far better than anything that had come before. Patients with *folie raisonnante* could be capable of lucid awareness and reasoning at the same time that they were insane.

Pinel discarded humoral and other outmoded theories, and instead looked to the environment and heredity as causative factors in mental disease.

WRONG! Everyone knows it's **animal magnetism!**

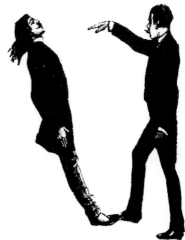

Franz Anton Mesmer (1734-1815), an Austrian physician, actually cured many patients with—you guessed it!—Mesmerism, which involved the laying on of hands and convincing the patient that the flow of animal magnetism was thereby corrected.

An English surgeon, **James Braid** (1795-1860) reworked Mesmer's method (calling it instead *hypnotism*) which he felt worked not because of any kind of 'magnetism' but by suggestion.

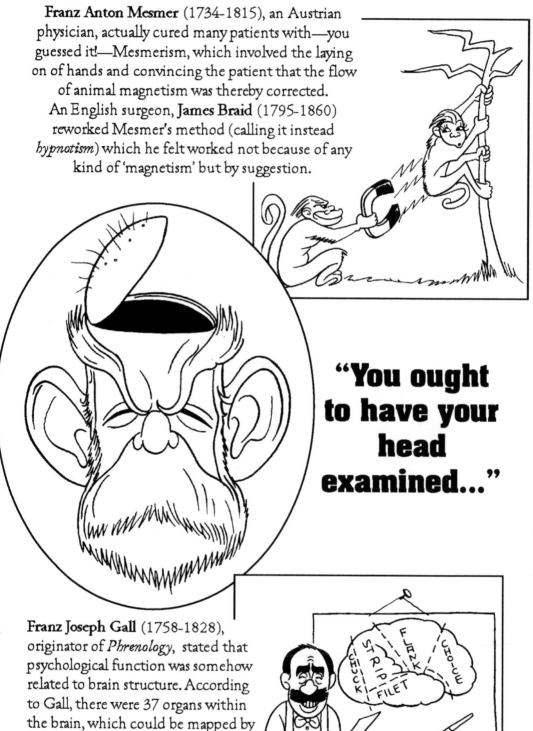

"You ought to have your head examined..."

Franz Joseph Gall (1758-1828), originator of *Phrenology*, stated that psychological function was somehow related to brain structure. According to Gall, there were 37 organs within the brain, which could be mapped by examining the surface of the head.

N ow, coming on up to the nineteenth century we find things really starting to get off the ground.

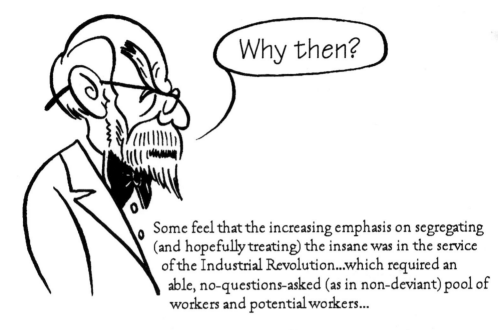

Why then?

Some feel that the increasing emphasis on segregating (and hopefully treating) the insane was in the service of the Industrial Revolution...which required an able, no-questions-asked (as in non-deviant) pool of workers and potential workers...

Classification (nosology) of psychiatric disorders was becoming more and more sophisticated. **Esquirol** (1782-1840), a French psychiatrist, furthered the cause of moral treatment, initiated formal training in psychiatry, invented the term 'hallucinations', differentiated these from illusions, and separated psychic from somatic causes of mental disorder.

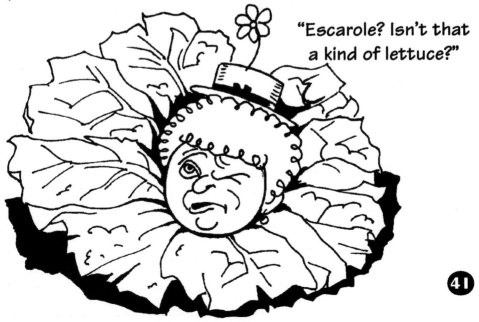

"Escarole? Isn't that a kind of lettuce?"

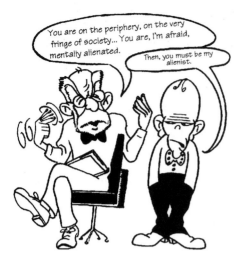

Jean Falret, another French psychiatrist of the time, documented what he called 'circular insanity' (known subsequently as *manic depression*), and coined the term 'mental alienation' to describe psychiatric illness.

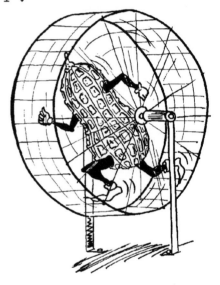

Like most things in life, the progression toward a rational humanist psychiatry wasn't always smooth or uphill [thumbs up and thumbs down]. Some French psychiatrists of the time espoused a theory of degeneration, claiming that insanity, alcoholism and other behavioral problems were passed along from one generation to the next, always worsening over the course of time. The Italian psychiatrist **Cesare Lombroso** (1836-1909) offered an evolutionary interpretation, viewing criminals as survivors of a primitive (degenerate) race. As the century ended, the degeneration theory eventually became discredited.

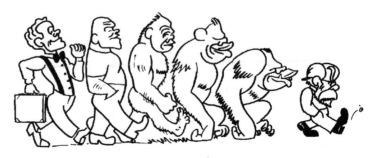

Cruel and unusual treatments of the time included dunking, castration, and the use of a particularly onerous device known as the 'Darwin chair.' The insane person was placed in this appliance and rotated until blood oozed from the the mouth, ears and nose; many therapeutic successes were reported as a result of its use. Patients at the Charite in Berlin were drenched with two hundred or more pails of water at a sitting.

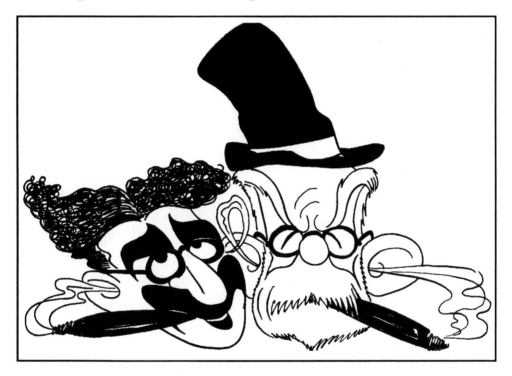

The *Commissioners of Lunacy* was established by two Acts of Parliament in 1845 to oversee the management of asylums in England.

•

In 1844 superintendants of U.S. asylums gathered together to form the Association of Medical Superintendants of American Institutions for the Insane (known today as the American Psychiatric Association.)

Meanwhile, back on the couch...

Johann **Reil's** (1759-1813) *Rhapsodies about the Application of Psychotherapy to Mental Disturbances* laid the foundation for modern psychotherapy.

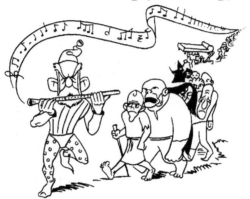

Another German physician, Wilhelm **Griesinger** (1817-1868) published *Mental Pathology and Therapeutics*, which emphasized the role of the brain in mental illness and set the stage for the development of neuro- and brain psychiatry. Griesinger stressed the importance of *both* heredity and upbringing in the genesis of mental illness; mental illness had multiple causes.

Griesinger: "INSANITY IS MERELY A SYMPTOM-COMPLEX OF VARIOUS ANOMALOUS STATES IN THE BRAIN."

These psychiatries attempt to correlate brain structure with function. (Bear in mind--oops, sorry!--the struggle, unresolved to this day, between 'somatic' and 'psychic' schools of thought.)

Brain psychiatry's cause was considerably furthered by the work of Alois **Alzheimer** (who described pathological changes in the brains of patients with the disease bearing his name) and by studies of *general paresis* (otherwise known as syphilis...) **Broca's** localization of the speech center to a certain area of the brain in 1861 further encouraged "speculative anatomists", who were attempting to match up specific brain areas with specific psychologic functions.

For literally thousands of years, psychiatric methods had to rely on anecdotal observation and speculation. Then came **Kraepelin**. Unlike his predecessors, Emil Kraepelin (German, 1855-1926) based his conclusions on the systematic clinical observation of thousands of patients...and came up with the following diagnostic scheme, still in use today:

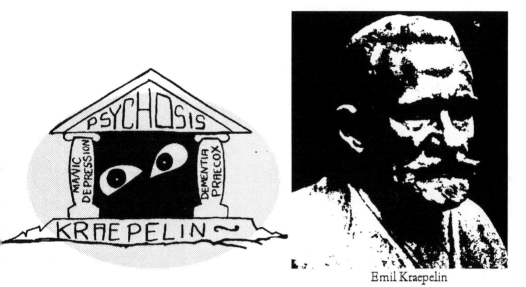

Emil Kraepelin

TWO CLASSES OF MAJOR PSYCHOSES:

(1) *manic depressive psychosis* (remember Falret's 'circular insanity'?-what goes around comes around!)

(2) *dementia praecox* (literally, early or premature dementia)

Kraepelin observed that the two major psychoses had vastly different outcomes. Whereas manic depressive illness usually remitted, with preservation of mental health and functioning between episodes, dementia praecox typically worsened over the course of time, leading ultimately to dementia. Three subgroups of praecox were noted: *catatonia, hebephrenia,* and *dementia paranoia.*

Kraepelin's work was further refined by the Swiss psychiatrist Eugen **Bleuler** (1857-1939), who substituted the term 'schizophrenia' for Kraepelin's 'dementia praecox'. Bleuler's schizophrenia was characterized by "the Three A's":

Autism: trapped in their own private world, schizophrenic patients have a peculiar inability to communicate with those around them.

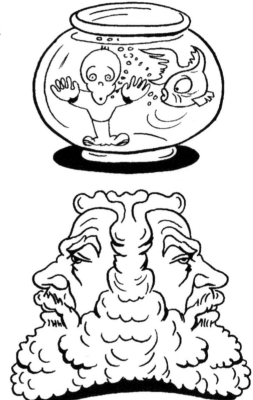

Ambivalence: schizophrenics typically waver back and forth, having extreme difficulty with decisions of any kind.

Associations: schizophrenic speech (and therefore thinking) is marked by 'loosening' of associations...the schizophrenic's thought will jump, or derail, making seemingly illogical leaps from one topic to another.

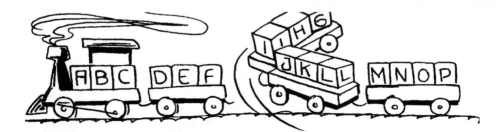

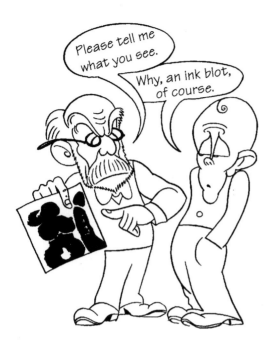

The ink blot test pioneered by **H. Rorschach** in 1921 helped amplify existing diagnostic methods

Meanwhile, back in the snakepit...

The response to the growing numbers of patients in asylums in the second half of the nineteenth century was a move from moral treatment to plain old custodialism. With increasing recognition that certain mental illness was treatable, however, short term psychiatric hospitalization became more available as an alternative.

The turn of the century ushered in heightened awareness of problems in the asylums, and a blossoming of new interventions in mental illness including psychiatric social work, and occupational and recreational therapy.

The work of **Adolph Meyer** (American, 1866-1950), helped consolidate this new approach. Meyer's emphasis was at once dynamic and synthetic: the patient became ill as a result of both internal and enironmental factors, and treatment needed to be holistic, targeted at both the individual and his social context.

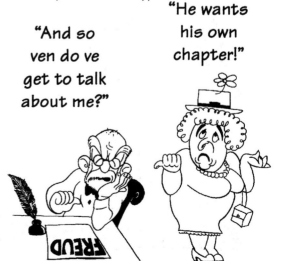

Let's follow the yellow pill road...

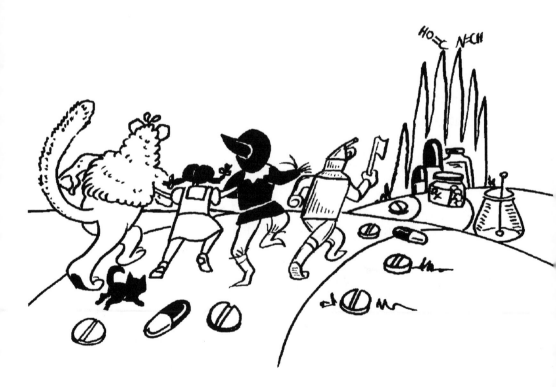

Should I see a shrink?

It is no longer fashionable to blame our problems on spirit possession, demons, voodoo, etc. (Although there are some who would disagree!)

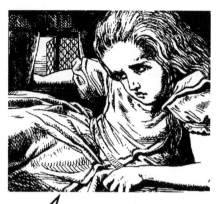

These days we are far more likely to attribute our difficulties to 'stress' or 'problems in living.' When people describe an inner source of distress, they may say that they feel 'nervous', 'depressed', or 'out of control.'

SPEAKING OF WHICH: WHAT EXACTLY IS A 'NERVOUS BREAKDOWN'?

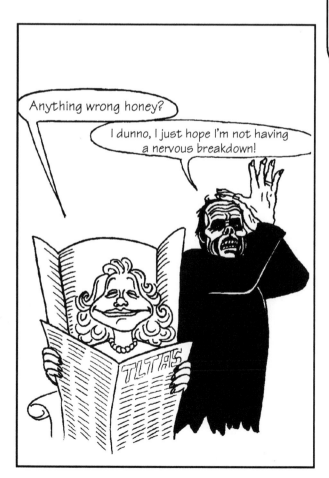

Anything wrong honey?

I dunno, I just hope I'm not having a nervous breakdown!

Answer: No such animal! 'Nervous breakdown' is a catch-all term that can mean depression, anxiety. inability to function from day to day, etc... No psychiatrist worth his salt uses this expression nowadays.

Typical responses to such distress include:

• watching and waiting, to see if the problem will disappear on its own;

• talking it over with friends and family, in an effort to identify and possibly eliminate the cause;

• 'self-medicating'--that is, attempting to make oneself feel better--with alcohol, drugs, sex, exercise, work, food, or shopping.

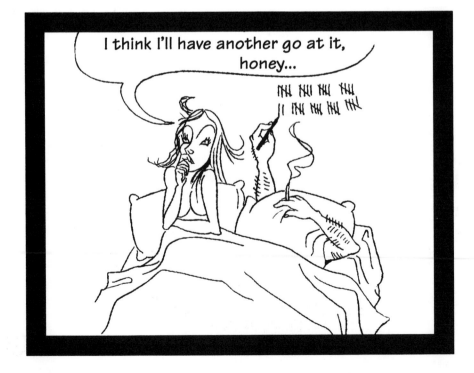

When none of these measures suffice; when one's relationships, work and social functioning are suffering as a result; then it may be reasonable to visit...a shrink.

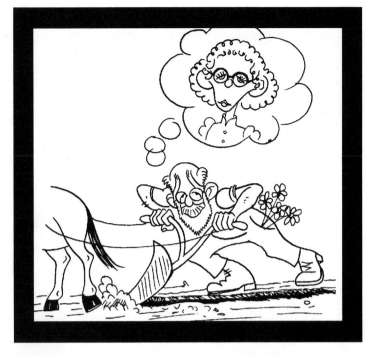

Sigmund Freud [1856-1939] defined mental health as 'the ability to work and love.'

Why do people become psychiatrists?

Interesting question. (Chances are, if you asked a psychiatrist, he or she would answer...with a question of their own!)

According to a recent informal survey of practitioners, it appears that some enter the field in order to understand themselves better, to work out their own unresolved conflicts and problems. Helping others do that may be a way of mastering old feelings of frustration and helplessness in the face of emotional pain.

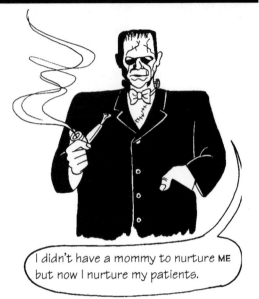

I didn't have a mommy to nurture ME but now I nurture my patients.

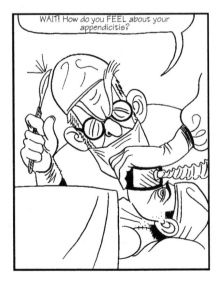

WAIT! How do you FEEL about your appendicitis?

Other psychiatrists knew all along that they wanted to be doctors, but became impressed at some point with the importance of the mind in determining outcomes in disease and health. Some felt that the extent of interpersonal contact available in general medicine was insufficient for them, and they wanted more in-depth dialogue or involvement with their patients.

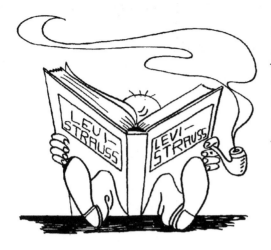

One of the major appeals of psychiatry is its humanistic (as opposed to strictly scientific) slant. In order to effectively treat his patients, the psychiatrist must be aware of the diverse social and political forces impacting them. The psychiatrist should be culturally as well as emotionally literate.

What do psychiatrists *do*?

Psychiatrists practice in a variety of settings, including offices, clinics (public and private), emergency rooms and hospital-based (inpatient) programs.

Contrary to popular belief, most psychiatrists' offices do *not* feature a couch. More likely you will be seated upright, face to face with the interviewing psychiatrist during your first consultation. He or she will be evaluating not only your stated reason for coming (your *chief complaint*), but a host of other factors as well.

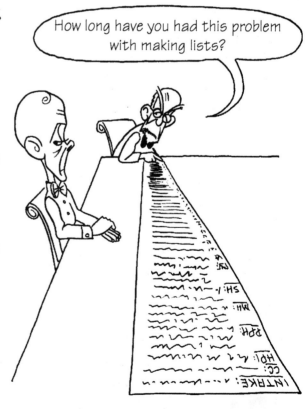

How long have you had this problem with making lists?

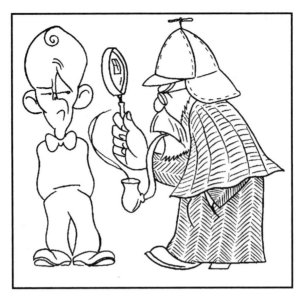

The doctor will be interested in your *general appearance*, your *relatedness* (as manifested by level of eye contact, body language, presence or absence of tension, guardedness), your *mood*, and in both the *form* and *content* of your speech. He or she will usually want to know about your sleep and eating patterns, and about the presence of any memory or language or calculation difficulties.

The psychiatrist will be particularly concerned about the *history* of the problem: When did it begin? Have you ever had a similar problem before? What kind of things alleviate the problem? What makes it worse? How has the problem affected your work and home life?

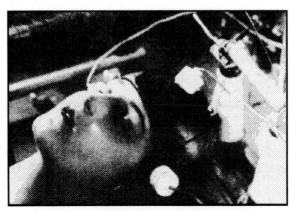

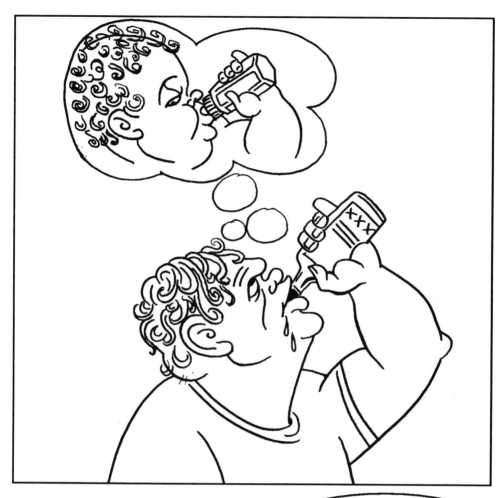

Of at least equal importance is the history of the individual who is seeking help. Where did you grow up? With whom, and under what circumstances? What was your earliest memory? Do any of your early experiences stand out as being particularly painful and/or memorable? Were there any significant early losses?

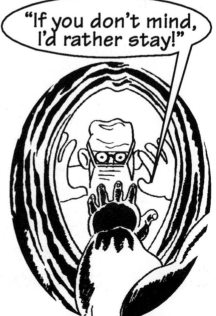

How did you do in school? Did you and do you have close friends? Love relationships? What kinds of attachments do you form to people? How is your sex life? Your fantasy life? What kinds of jobs have you held and how long for? What are your ambitions?

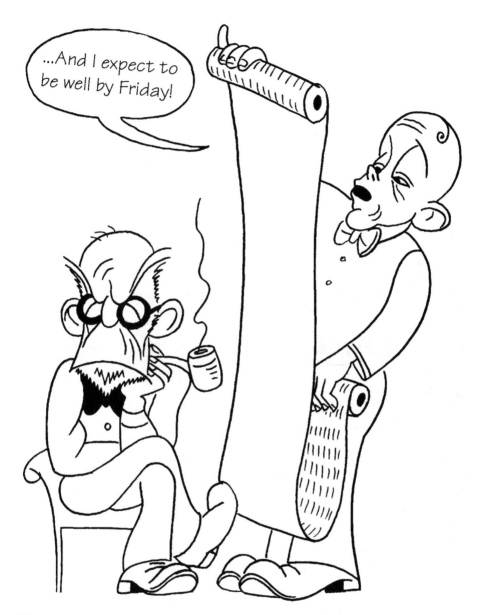

This list is by no means exhaustive. Depending on his or her approach, the psychiatrist may conduct a fairly open-ended interview, leaving it up to the patient to fill in the relevant details, or may instead pursue a more systematic formalized evaluation. In either case, it is important during the initial session(s) for the potential patient to fully express his concerns, his questions, and his expectations of treatment.

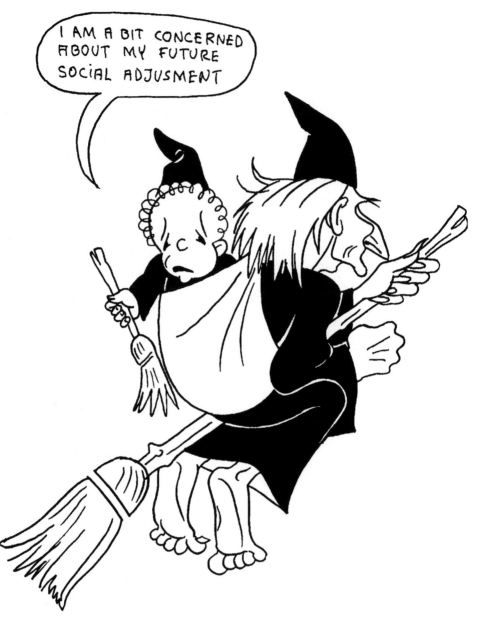

You'll notice how much of an emphasis this kind of evaluation places on *individual* relationships, interactions, and losses. In fact, most of the psychotherapy practiced these days focuses on problematic early relationships—with people. Some would argue that the larger current relationships—our relationships with our society, our culture, and our environment—are thereby short-changed. How do we know that living in a crazy problem-riddled society doesn't make us crazy too?

The evaluation process should be reciprocal. The psychiatric consumer should likewise be evaluating the doctor, along the following lines: Do I feel comfortable with this person? Is this someone I feel I could trust? Does he or she appear generally interested in me, in what brought me to the consultation room? Am I reasonably satisfied with the arrangements the doctor is suggesting, including frequency of visits, length of sessions, fee structure? Can I expect to benefit from the proposed therapy? How? What alternative treatments exist for my problem?

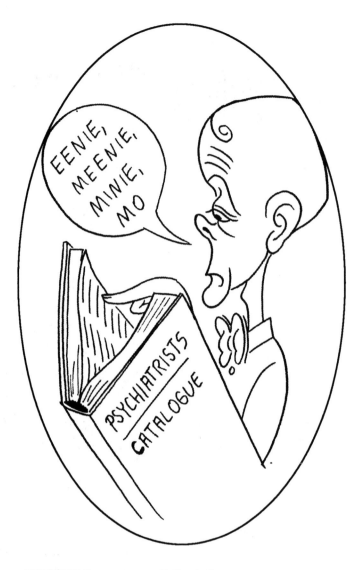

The psychiatric consumer should be an INFORMED consumer:

By comparison shopping (the potential patient may wish to interview one or more other psychiatrists before committing to a particular one); by reading and information gathering from libraries, television, and news media; by speaking to other individuals who have been treated for similar problems.

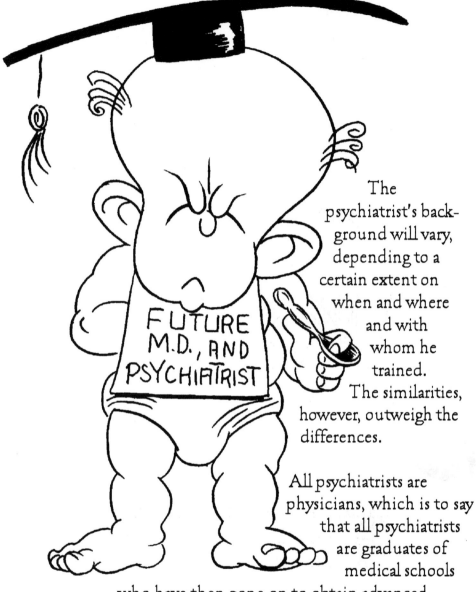

The psychiatrist's background will vary, depending to a certain extent on when and where and with whom he trained.

The similarities, however, outweigh the differences.

All psychiatrists are physicians, which is to say that all psychiatrists are graduates of medical schools who have then gone on to obtain advanced training in their chosen field (psychiatry.) This usually takes the form of four additional years in a psychiatric residency program, located in or near a teaching hospital so that the resident can have access to patients in multiple settings.

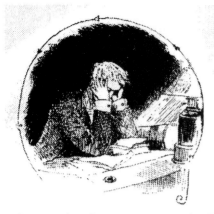

The psychiatric residency typically includes a year of hospital medicine, including obligatory nights 'on-call' (the intention here being to supplement the psychiatrist-in-training's medical background with an exhaustive, if not exhausting, clinical experience); extensive exposure to hospitalized psychiatric patients, who tend to be more severely ill and often require overlapping treatment approaches, including medication, psychotherapy, and social interventions; emergency room work, which hones the trainee's ability to deal with crises, and to recognize and treat a host of illnesses on an urgent basis; consultation/liaison visits with medically hospitalized patients who may also be struggling with problems like depression, anxiety, and loss (the challenge for the resident here being to separate 'medical' from 'emotional' illness, and to serve not only as healer for the patient but as teacher and treatment coordinator for hospital personnel working with the patient); psychotherapy with both hospitalized and ambulatory patients, conducted under the supervision of more senior psychiatrists; and elective time, which can be devoted to research or additional work in any of the areas mentioned above.

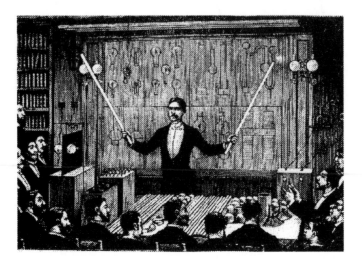

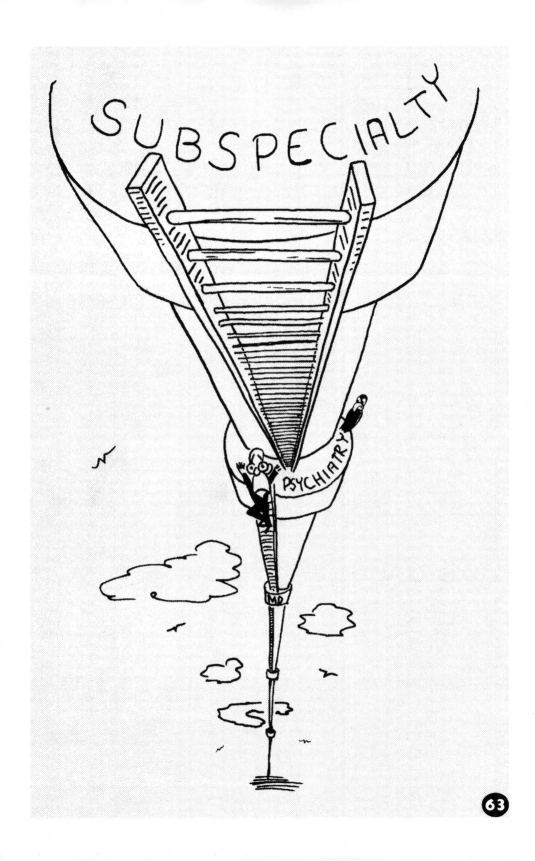

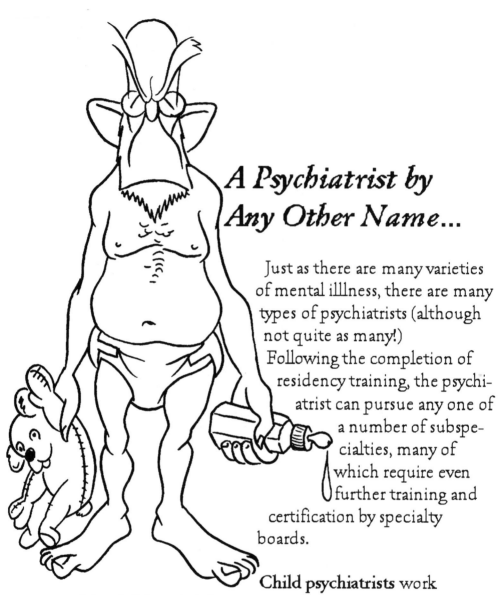

A Psychiatrist by Any Other Name...

Just as there are many varieties of mental illllness, there are many types of psychiatrists (although not quite as many!)
Following the completion of residency training, the psychiatrist can pursue any one of a number of subspecialties, many of which require even further training and certification by specialty boards.

Child psychiatrists work with...children (adolescents, too.)

This type of work requires certain modifications of clinical technique. Psychiatrists who work with children must be willing to literally get down on the floor with their patients. Children will often be able to dramatize inner and family conflicts by means of drawings and play.

Aging populations are served by *geropsychiatrists,* who have particular expertise with problems like dementia and grieving among the elderly. [The elderly, by the way, are the fastest growing segment of many populations these days.]

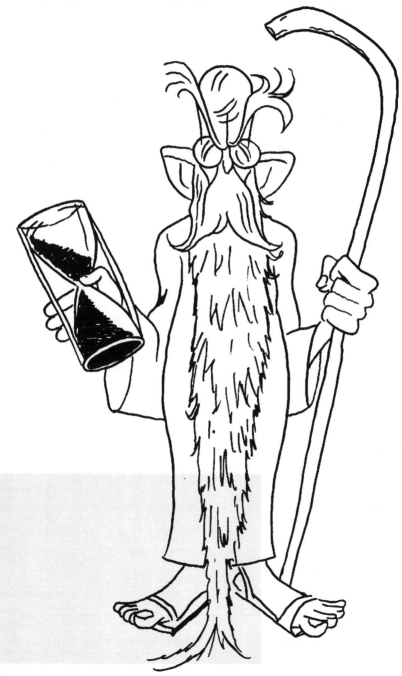

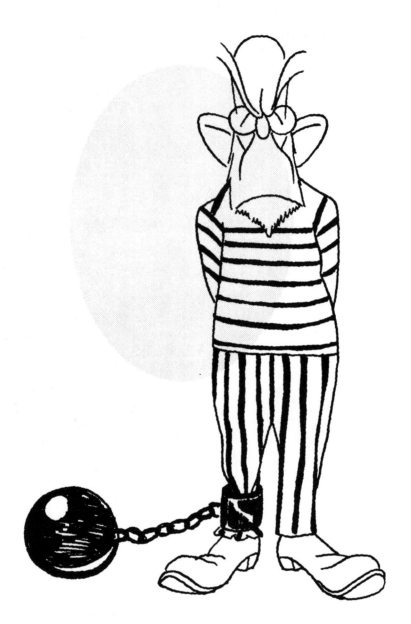

F*orensic psychiatrists* work with incarcerated patients and are often called upon as expert witnesses in such matters as competence to stand trial and other sensitive medical/ethical decisions.

The special needs of alcoholics and other addicts are addressed by *addiction psychiatrists*, who treat individuals with chemical and other dependencies. In recent years, addiction psychiatry has attempted to extend its domain to other 'compulsive' or 'appetitive' behaviors such as gambling, overeating, shopping, and even sex.

"You mean there's such a thing as too much sex?"

PSYCHOPHARMACOLOGISTS may be able to offer more sophisticated approaches to the medication treatment of mental disorders. Although there are exceptions, many psychopharmacologists avoid talking therapies, sticking instead to the prescription of drugs.

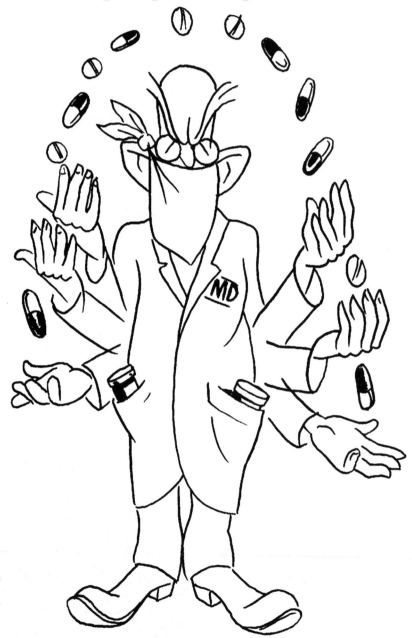

What can I expect when I see one?

Psychiatrists differ in their approaches to patients' problems. Some will stick to a strictly biologic (medication-oriented) approach, while others will be more interested in helping you to better understand your motivations and the 'unconscious' roots of your difficulties.

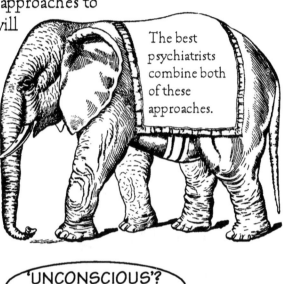

The best psychiatrists combine both of these approaches.

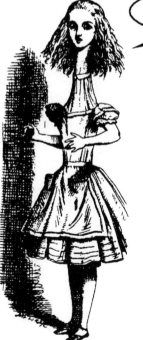

'UNCONSCIOUS'? What's that?

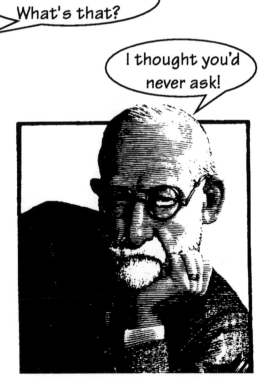

I thought you'd never ask!

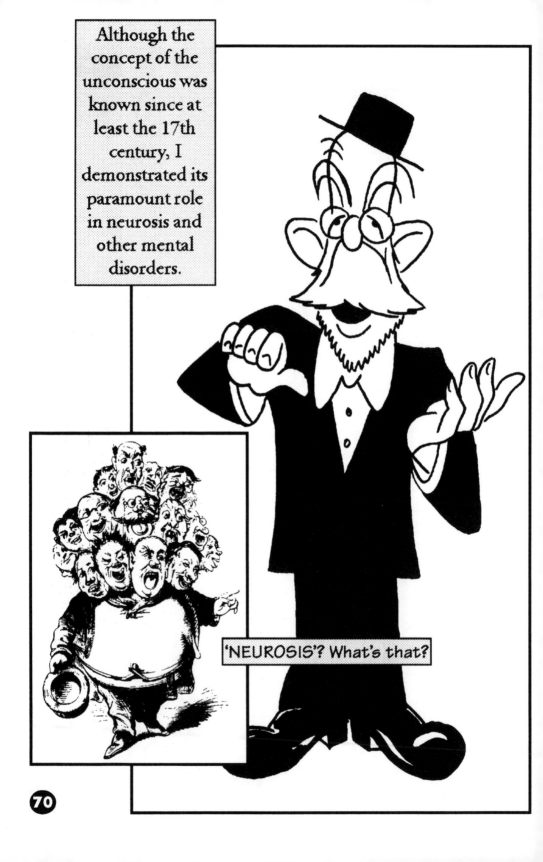

Although the concept of the unconscious was known since at least the 17th century, I demonstrated its paramount role in neurosis and other mental disorders.

'NEUROSIS'? What's that?

Doctors in the latter part of the 18th century had to come up with a name for problems which had no apparent physical cause, such as preoccupation with imagined illness (*hypochondriasis*) and complaints of paralysis, numbness or fainting (*hysteria*). These were termed **neuroses**.

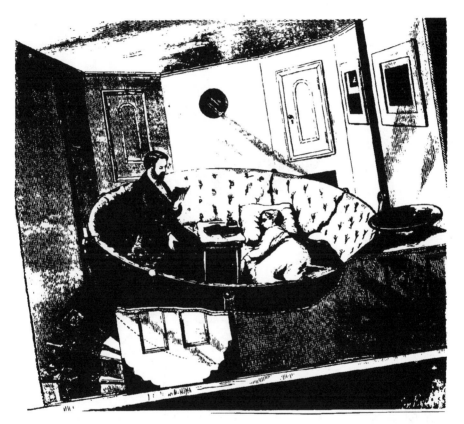

Hysterics were almost always women (although Freud, to his credit, later reported that men could also suffer from hysteria.) Unfortunately, theories of flawed female anatomy (in this case, 'ovarian pressure') were still highly favored at the time, and were used to justify thousands upon thousands of unnecessary surgical procedures on female patients.

Jean Martin **Charcot** (1825-1893), director of the
Salpetriere, pioneered the use of hypnosis in the
treatment of his hysterical patients.

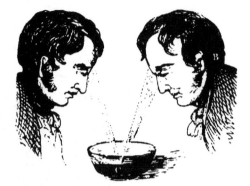

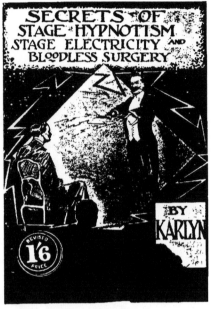

Later, Hippolyte Marie **Bernheim**
(1837-1919) showed that the healing force at work in hypnotism was
nothing other than
suggestion.

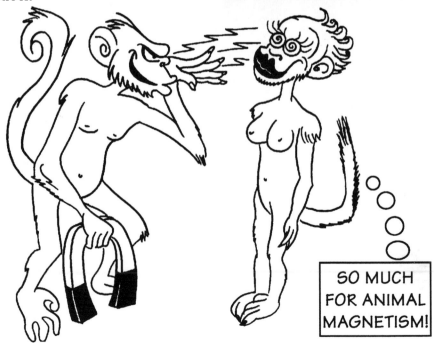

SO MUCH
FOR ANIMAL
MAGNETISM!

Pierre **Janet** (1859-1947) found that painful experiences, once forgotten ('repressed'), could cause neurotic symptoms; and even more important, he found that uncovering these traumatic memories ('catharsis') with hypnosis could lead to cure.

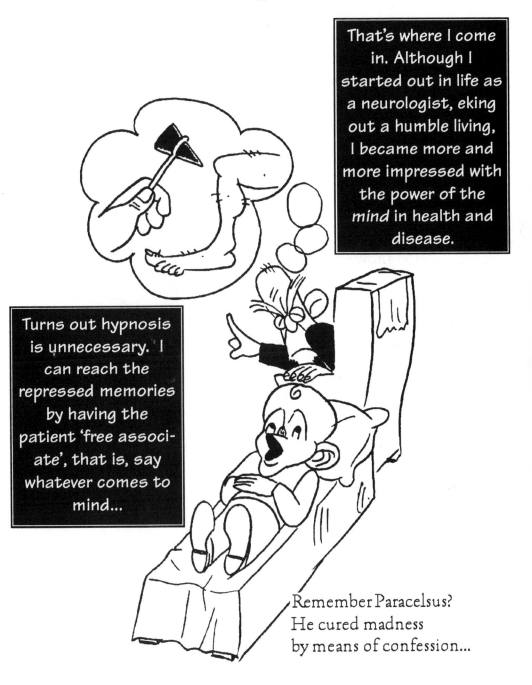

That's where I come in. Although I started out in life as a neurologist, eking out a humble living, I became more and more impressed with the power of the mind in health and disease.

Turns out hypnosis is unnecessary. I can reach the repressed memories by having the patient 'free associate', that is, say whatever comes to mind...

Remember Paracelsus? He cured madness by means of confession...

Sigmund Freud studied with Charcot, was familiar with the work of Janet and Bernheim, and eventually collaborated with Joseph **Breuer**. Their *Studies on Hysteria* (1895) described *conversion* (i.e., painful memories are 'converted' into paralysis or numbness) symptoms among hysterics.

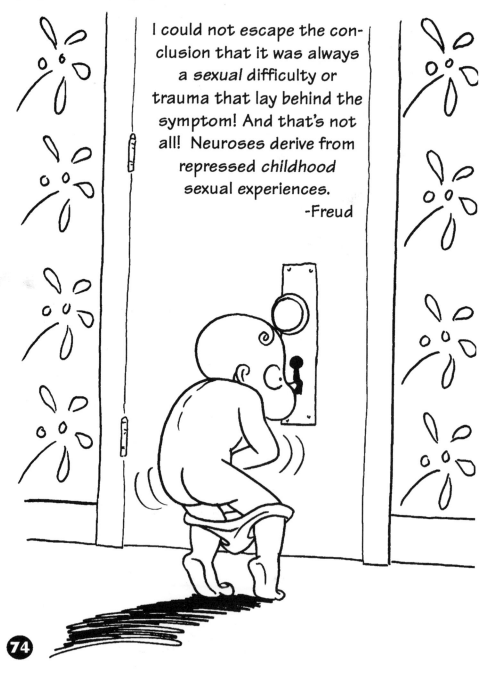

I could not escape the conclusion that it was always a sexual difficulty or trauma that lay behind the symptom! And that's not all! Neuroses derive from repressed *childhood* sexual experiences.
-Freud

This was too much for Breuer. Freud had gone too far. Besides which, Breuer was stuck on physiological explanations, while Freud was moving more and more toward purely psychological explanations of disordered behavior.

But where do these repressed memories go?

Elementary, my dear Alice. Into the Unconscious, of course!

According to Freud, our day-to-day waking awareness is but the tip of the iceberg of the psyche. Beneath this conscious level lies a nearly limitless depth of *drives* (like sex and aggression), feelings, and memories.

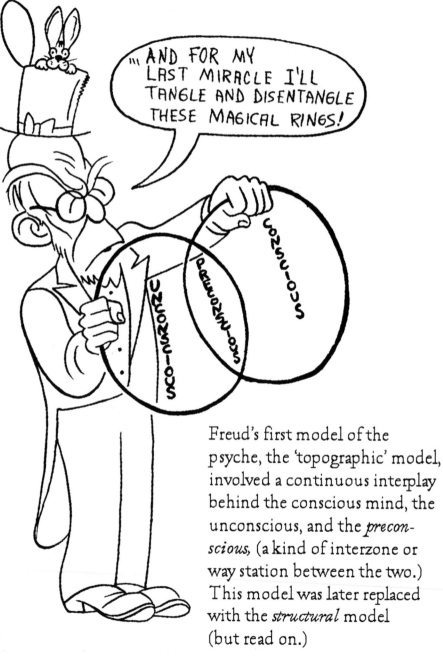

"...AND FOR MY LAST MIRACLE I'LL TANGLE AND DISENTANGLE THESE MAGICAL RINGS!

UNCONSCIOUS

PRECONSCIOUS

CONSCIOUS

Freud's first model of the psyche, the 'topographic' model, involved a continuous interplay behind the conscious mind, the unconscious, and the *preconscious*, (a kind of interzone or way station between the two.) This model was later replaced with the *structural* model (but read on.)

Unconscious material erupts to the surface in the form of dreams, *parapraxes* ('Freudian slips', memory lapses) and during the process of free association. Further, unresolved feelings about important figures from the patient's past are revealed in the patient's *transference* toward the doctor. The therapeutic work of interpreting these Freud termed *psychoanalysis*.

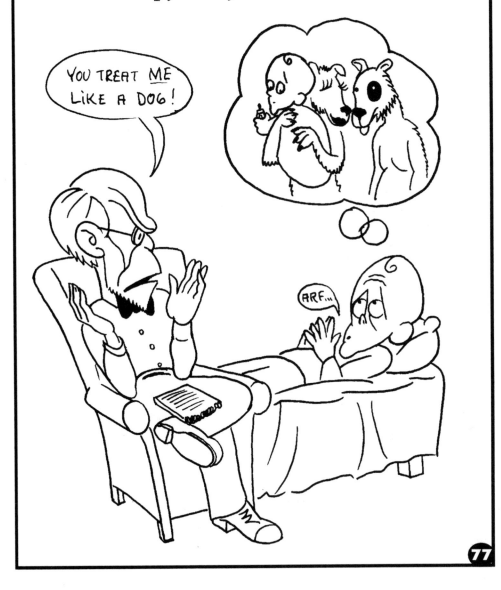

Psychoanalysis is a time- and labor- and wallet-intensive pursuit. The patient is expected to spend three to five one hour sessions a week with the analyst, recalling memories and free associating and eventually developing a *transference neurosis* to the doctor which the doctor can eventually connect to the patient's past. (Psychotics and those with severe personality disorders, incapable of forming such an emotional attachment to the doctor, were considered unworkable.) Freudian analysts tend to be reserved, limiting their comments to patients in an effort to promote the transference neurosis.

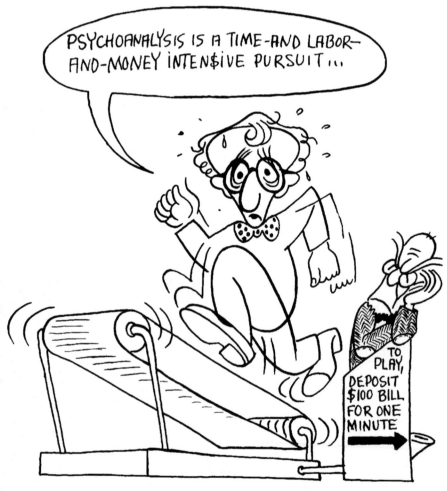

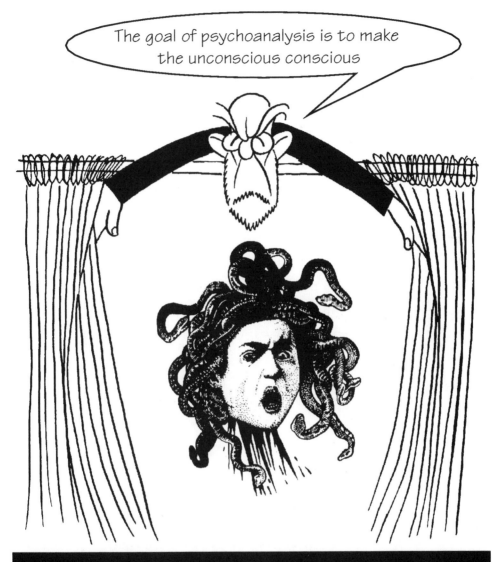

The Freudian inner world is densely populated by fantasies, unresolved conflicts, and perhaps chiefly by 'unneutralized' sexual (and aggressive) strivings: Freud's *drive theory*. Hints of these strivings take the form of ubiquitous *phallic* and vaginal symbols in dreams and patients' associations. Neurotics are doomed to live out a *repetition compulsion* (a pressing need to repeat behaviors) of *repressed* (forgotten) painful events until these are worked out in therapy.

TAKE NOTE: this is a very pessimistic attitude toward human nature. According to Dr. Freud, we are irrational creatures, driven by largely unconscious urges to fornicate and destroy...

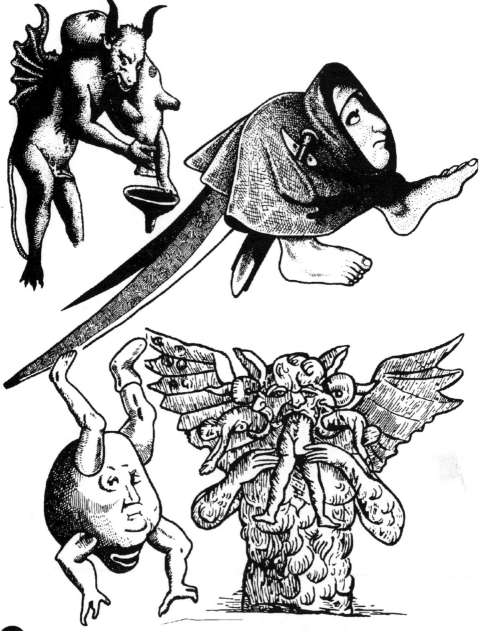

In the Freudian domain, libido (sex drive) is king.

Infancy and early childhood are dominated by sexuality. The young boy wants to sleep with his mother and kill his father (*Oedipus complex*). At the same time he fears major reprisal from Dad (*castration anxiety*.)

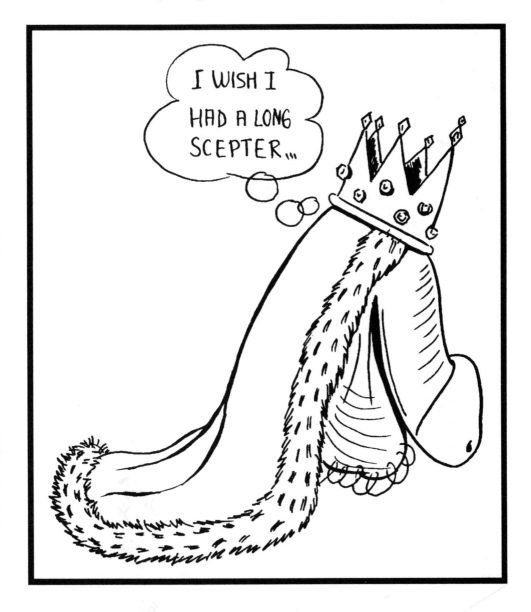

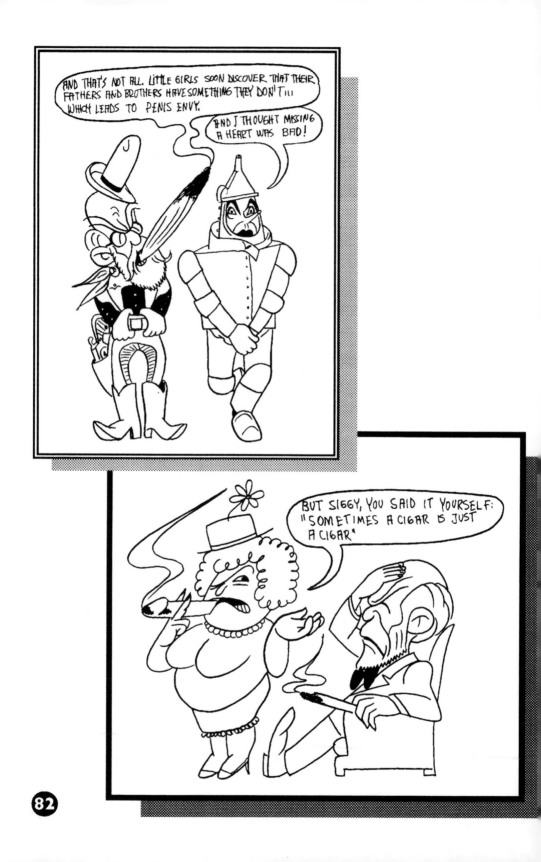

82

The child's sexual development passes through typical stages. The infant's world is centered around the mouth (**oral stage**.) All the good things in life, like warm milk and mother's breast, are experienced orally. Later, the child becomes very concerned with his bowels (**anal stage**), and in fact treasures his 'productions' as his very first creative efforts in life.

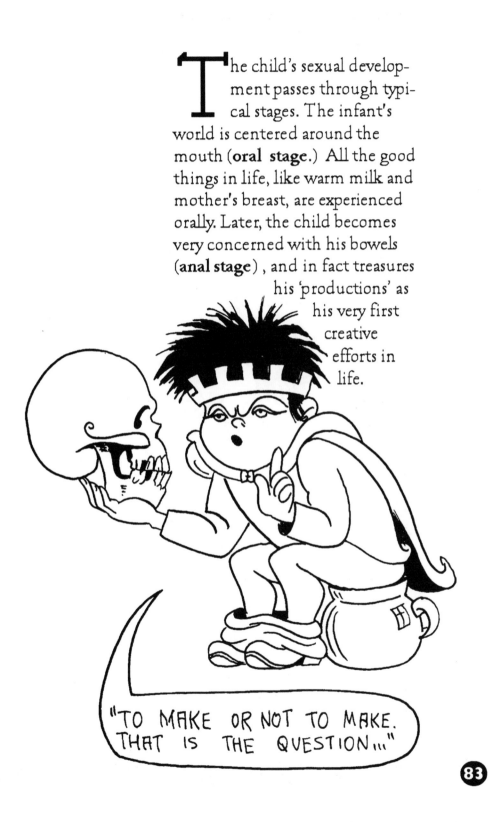

"TO MAKE OR NOT TO MAKE. THAT IS THE QUESTION..."

T his is succeeded in turn by the so-called **phallic stage**—
not to be confused with the final and most mature
stage, the **genital stage**, featuring the relocation of
sexual interest from the mouth and anus and other body parts
exclusively to the genitals. It is only at this stage that one is
capable of 'mature' heterosexual erotic love. (By this account,
only vaginal orgasm in women is healthy; clitoral orgasm is
considered immature, not fully 'grown up.')

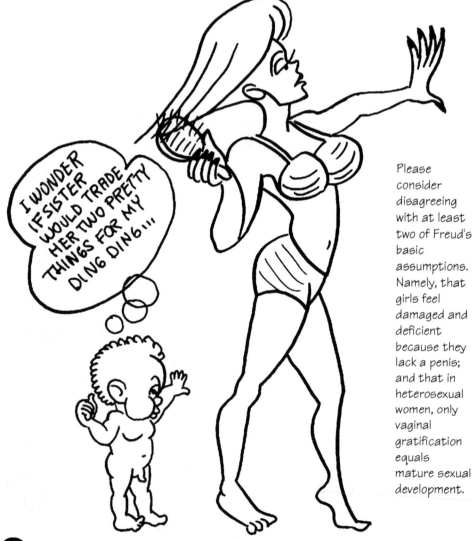

Please consider disagreeing with at least two of Freud's basic assumptions. Namely, that girls feel damaged and deficient because they lack a penis; and that in heterosexual women, only vaginal gratification equals mature sexual development.

According to Freud, the journey to 'mature' (i.e. genital) sexuality is fraught with danger.

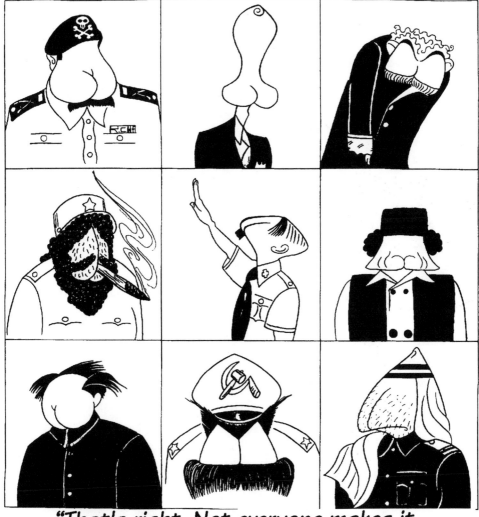

"That's right. Not everyone makes it. We all got stuck along the way."

I ndividuals may become *fixated* at any stage or during stress may *regress* from a more mature stage to an earlier one. 'Oral' personalities continue to experience the world largely through their mouths, via overeating, alcoholism, or drug addiction; 'anal' characters are said to be stingy, overly concerned with details and control. *Paraphilias* (perversions such as fetishism, voyeurism, exhibitionism, sadomasochism) are said to result from incomplete sexual development, where the erotic interest focuses on a particular body part or activity rather than on the partner as a whole.

Freud's later *structural* model, involving ego, id, and superego, is the one that is widely recognized today. The **ego** is (or should be) the executive branch of the psyche, using reason and conscious planning to preserve and protect the individual. The **superego**, derived from the child's 'identifications' with authority figures such as parents and teachers, performs an essentially judicial function, rewarding the individual with praise for 'good' behavior and meting out guilt and remorse for 'bad.' The **id**, operating largely beyond conscious awareness, lobbies and occasionally legislates for the drives, toward the expression of libido and aggression.

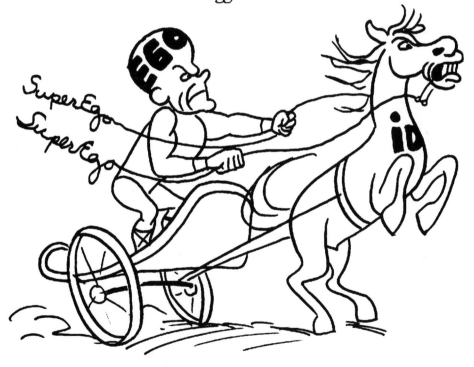

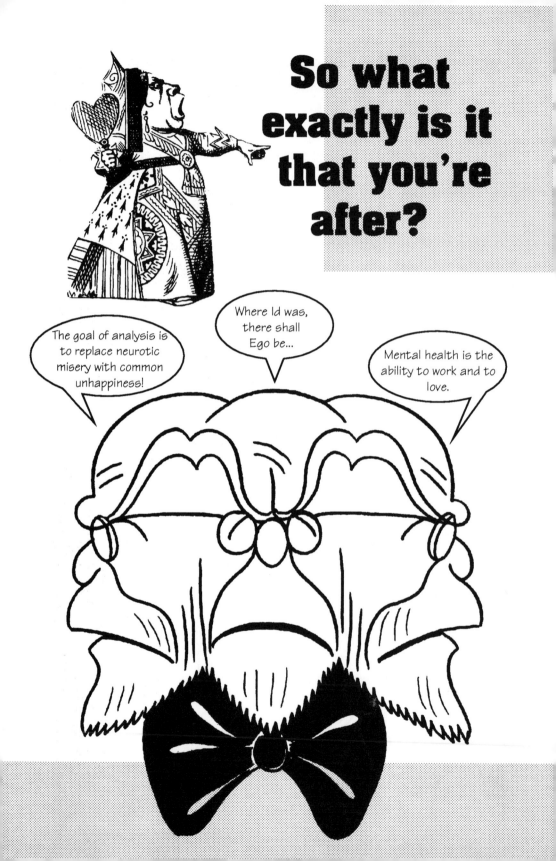

No doubt about it, Freud's contribution
was enormous. In addition to the above, he
described the role of **defense mechanisms** such as
*projection, denial, repression, rationalization, humor,
sublimation,* and *altruism* in the psychic 'economy';
posited a death instinct, *thanatos,* which was opposed to
the life instinct, or *eros;* and used psychoanalytic concepts
to explain not only the dynamics of depression
(in *Mourning and Melancholia*) but religion, which he
strenuously opposed (*The Future of an Illusion,*) and the
origins of art (essay on Michelangelo) and civilization
(*Civilization and Its Discontents, Totem and Taboo.*)

Freud's impact was indelible.
Humanity could never again
view itself as wholly rational. Darker
unconscious forces played themselves
out in man. Words and events had
deeper *meanings*.

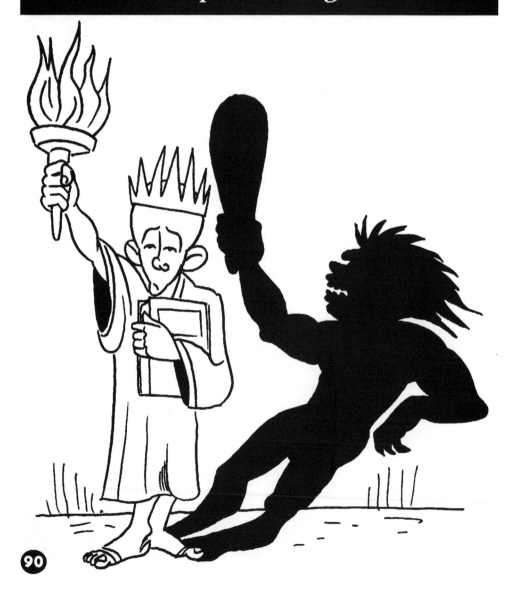

WHAT HAPPENED NEXT? HOW DID WE GET FROM THERE TO HERE?

Psychoanalysis became a *movement*.

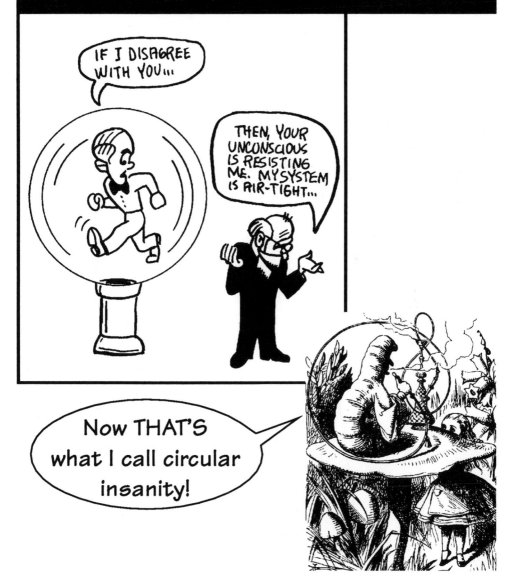

Freud's students became authorities in their own right.

Carl Jung [1876 - 1961] for example, one of the master's most favored disciples, eventually broke with Freud to found *analytic psychology*. His work on personality types (*introvert* vs. *extrovert*) was highly influential for decades. Jung felt that mental life was organized into *archetypes*, basic categories that determined human behavior and outlook and ambitions. His approach was a quasi-mystical, or spiritual, one: each of us participates in the *collective unconscious* which is a kind of group soul or psychic switchboard which links up the individual via his or her unconscious to humanity as a whole.

Sexuality is *not* everything! Man strives for self-knowledge.

Otto Rank insisted that *birth trauma*—the painful passage from the supposed safety of the womb through the birth canal into the harsh light of day—was crucial in understanding neurosis.

NO WAY JOSÉ!

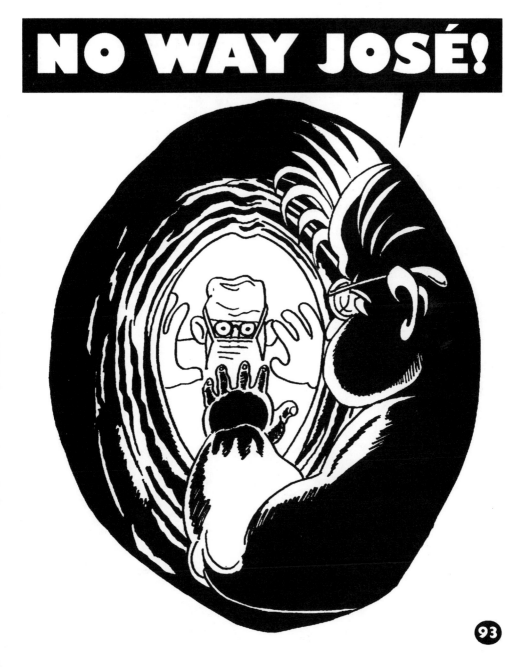

Freud's daughter **Anna Freud** (whom, incidentally, he analyzed) wrote extensively on defense mechanisms in her book *Ego and the Mechanisms of Defense.*

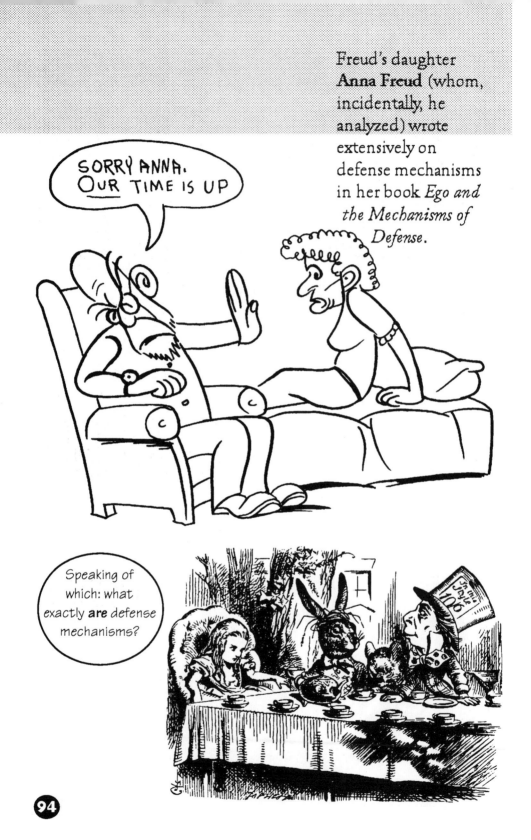

SORRY ANNA. OUR TIME IS UP

Speaking of which: what exactly **are** defense mechanisms?

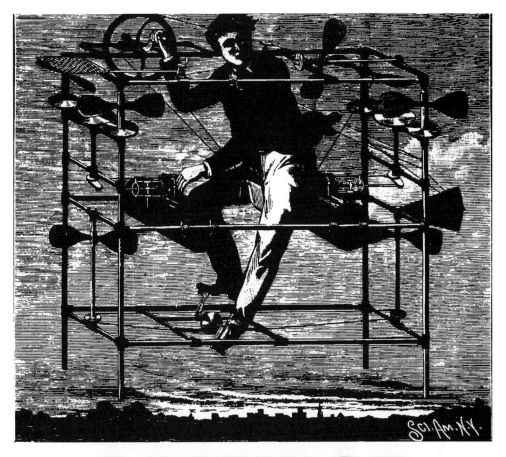

DEFENSE MECHANISMS

are means that the ego has at its disposal to deal with threatening or anxiety-provoking situations:

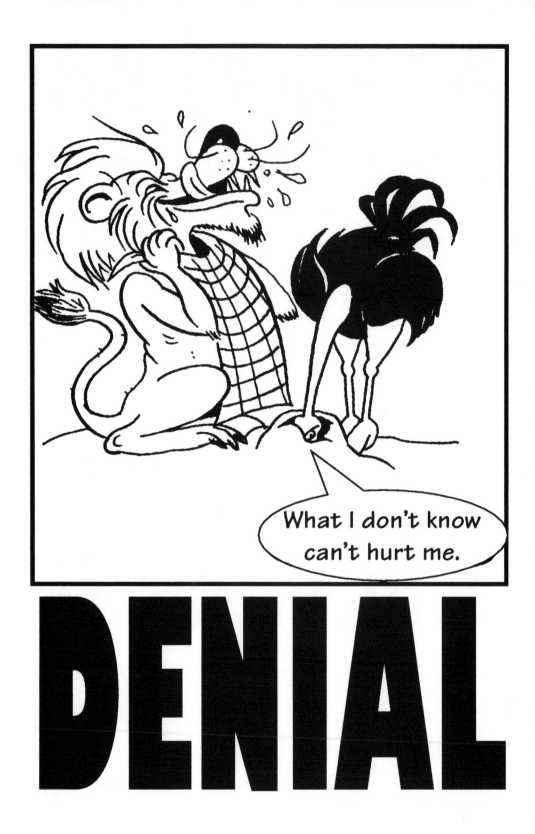

DENIAL

PROJECTION

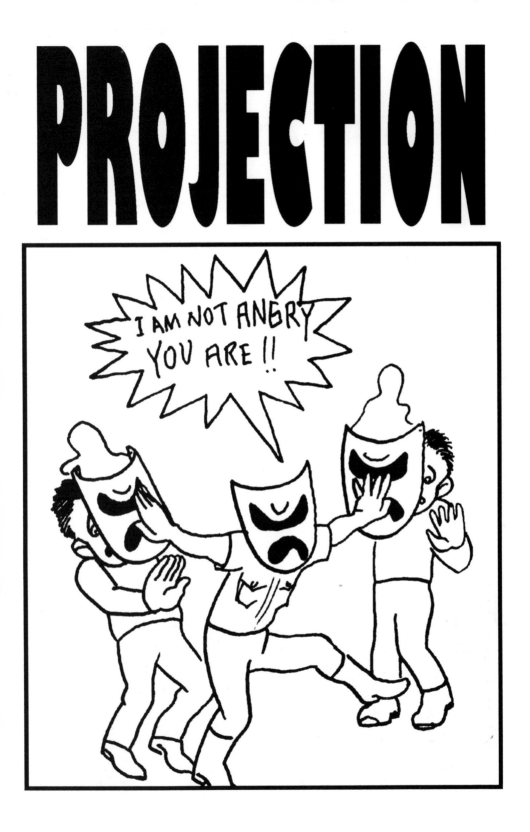

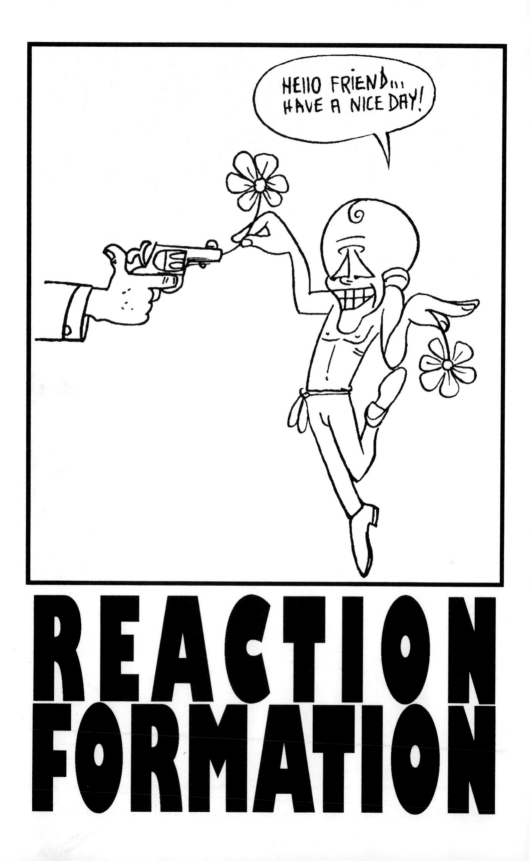

HUMOR

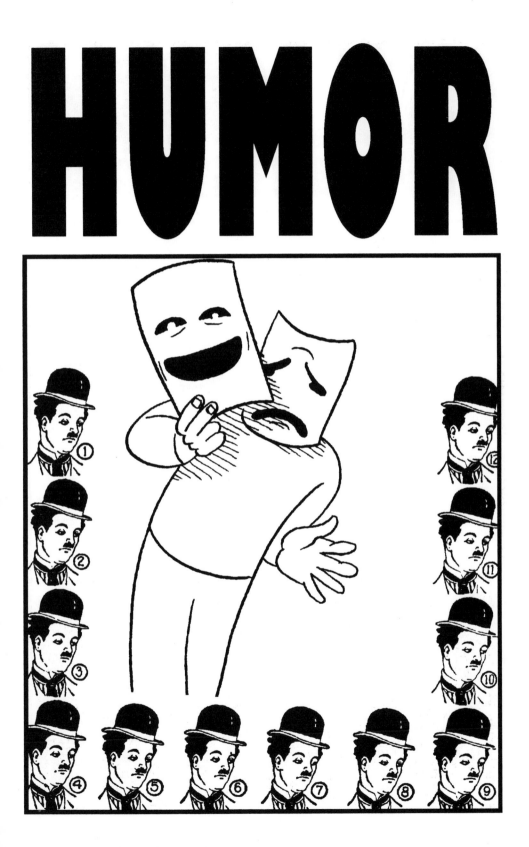

DISPLACEMENT

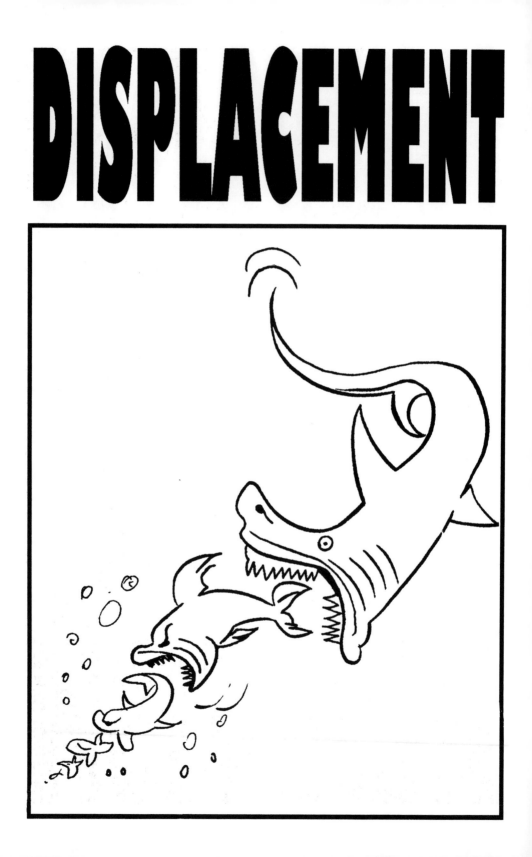

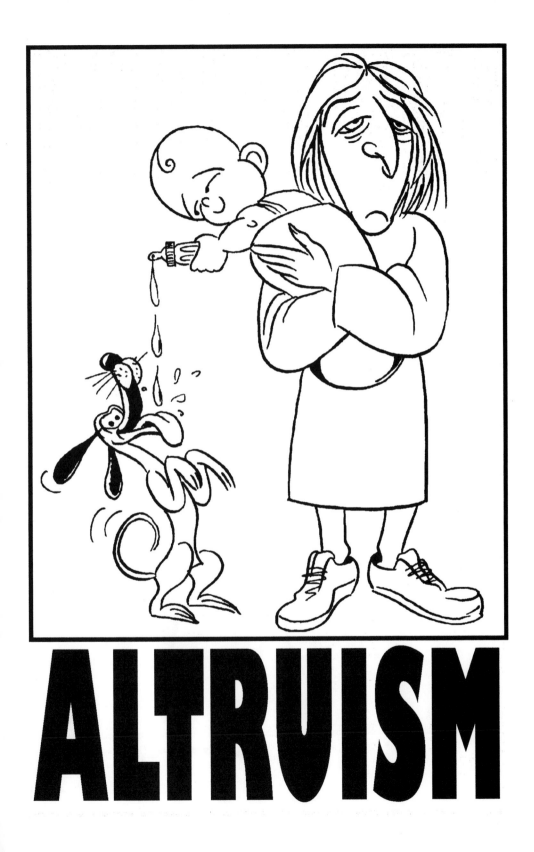

ALTRUISM

RATIONALIZATION

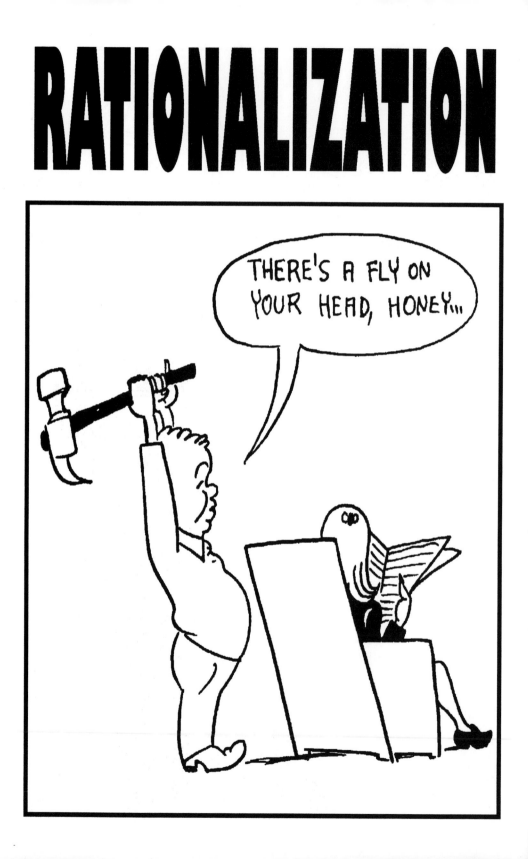

Wilhelm Reich described the effect of trauma and psychic conflict on body musculature. According to Reich, neurotics wear *character armor*, habitual postures and body language that prevent natural energies from flowing. Reich's prescription? One or more sessions in the *orgone box*, which he claimed had remarkable restorative effects.

Reader Quiz:

WHAT'S WRONG WITH THIS PICTURE?

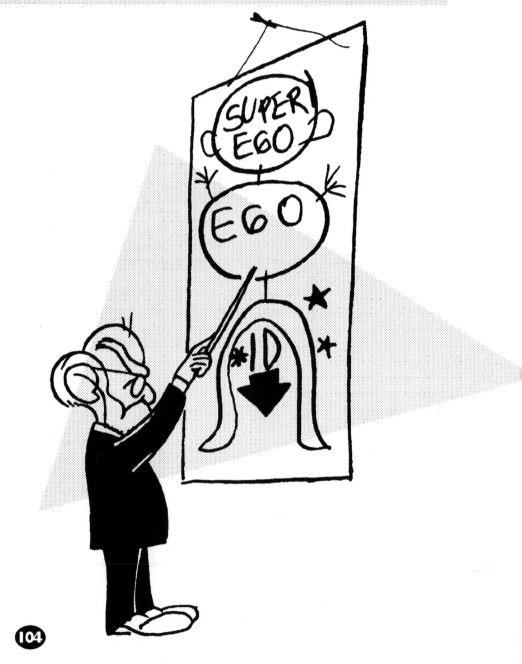

Answers:

(1) The emphasis on sexuality could be an artifact of Freud's use of cocaine (for which he had an admitted fondness.) Cocaine is known to provoke intensely erotic feelings in its users.

(2) Freudian dogma is unabashedly individualist. Psychic life begins and ends with the individual. There is little sense of interaction, of the effect that one person has on another.

THIS GUY'S GOT SEX ON HIS BRAIN. BETTER GO EASY ON THE COCAINE...

(3) There's no proof that the method works. (4) Freud et al's conclusions are based on a very narrow sample, namely bourgeois Victorian Viennese. (5) The doctrine itself is by its own standards immature (fixated at a narcissistic stage of development.) If the goal of healthy development is empathic relationship with others, then psychoanalysis, with its exclusive focus on the individual psyche (or as some would claim, on the bellybutton), its complete inattention to social issues and action, fails the test.

THE NEO-FREUDIANS

In time, the Freudian canon was expanded and revised. *Object relationists* like D.W. Winnicott, Melanie Klein, Edith Jacobson, Michael Balint, and Margaret Mahler paid more and more attention to *relational* issues like separation and attachment in infancy. Psychological maturation meant increasing awareness of and interaction with 'objects' (other people.) Life was, at least ideally, a series of evolving dialogues that supported and nurtured the individual.

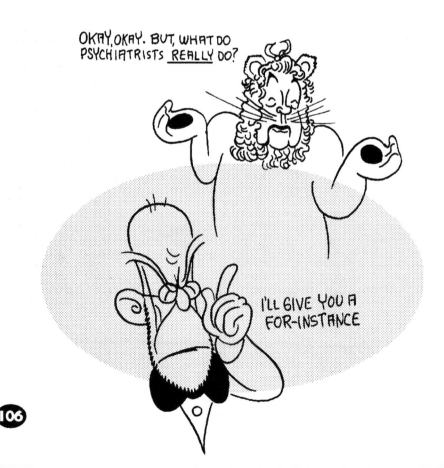

OKAY, OKAY. BUT, WHAT DO PSYCHIATRISTS REALLY DO?

I'LL GIVE YOU A FOR-INSTANCE

One day in November 1912* I was meeting with Jung and some other colleagues...and I fell into a dead faint. Naturally I was astonished at my loss of control. If I had gone to an analyst—but naturally I didn't, since *I* founded psychoanalysis and was happier analyzing myself, anyway—he would have helped me remember that it was in this very same hotel room that my relationship with my former colleague Fliess ended. Perhaps this incident has something to do with my relationship with my father... and with my feelings toward men in general!

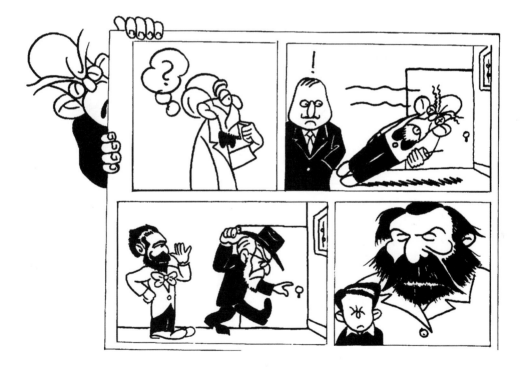

*note: this is a true story

Ah, that's nothing. My story's much better! Anyway, listen: One day, a day just like any other day, I'm coming home and what do you think I find? I find my husband, dead in bed, cold and stiff as a fish out of water. A heart attack. Weeks later, after all the shock and tumult are gone, I find I don't want to leave the apartment. I feel strange, guilty, as if I was somehow responsible for what happened. I can't sleep, I can't eat.

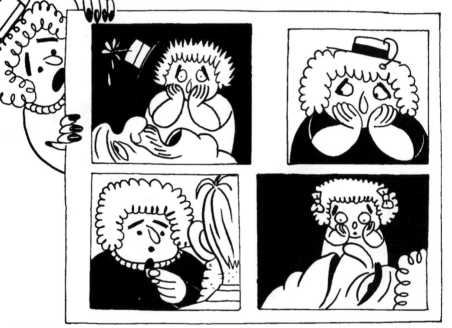

My friends say to me, *Rose, you're depressed. You need to see a doctor.* I hem and I haw, I put up a fight: Who wouldn't get depressed, walking into a scene like that? Well, finally I give in, I see this *psychiatrist,* and what do you think we do? We talk. And talk and talk and talk some more. He gives me some medication, an 'antidepressant' he calls it, and what do you know? In a couple of weeks I'm feeling much better, I'm getting out of the house...and he helps me realize that part of the reason for my terrible reaction was that *I lost my mother in almost exactly the same way.*

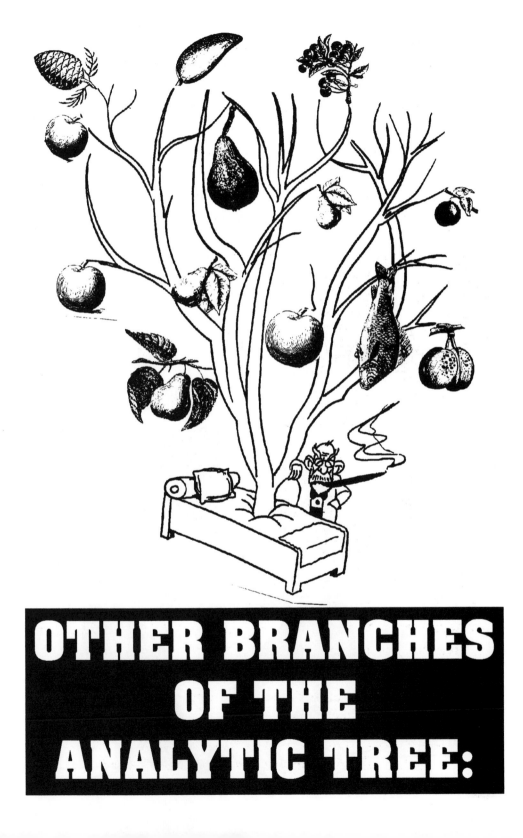

OTHER BRANCHES OF THE ANALYTIC TREE:

Alfred Adler, a contemporary of Freud, stressed the central role of the infant's helplessness; this led to the *inferiority complex* and subsequent strivings to achieve superiority and mastery. Unlike Freud, Adler insisted that the inner psychological world was not a mere 'knee-jerk' response to external events, but was in fact *created* by the individual.

Because he felt that patients' 'inner' life was hidden, i.e., unavailable for study, the American analyst **Harry Stack Sullivan** emphasized the role of cultural factors and **observable** interactions in his approach. *Freud's 'id psychology', based on instinct, was very much a product of turn-of-the-century Europe. Sullivan's psychology, with its focus on the ego, on the here-and-now, perhaps reflected the greater optimism of its American context.* In this view, Oedipal conflict and penis envy were not inevitable outcomes of normal development. Analysts could learn more by abandoning preconceived notions like 'aggressive drive' and simply *observing* their patients. The analyst's silence was not necessarily helpful.

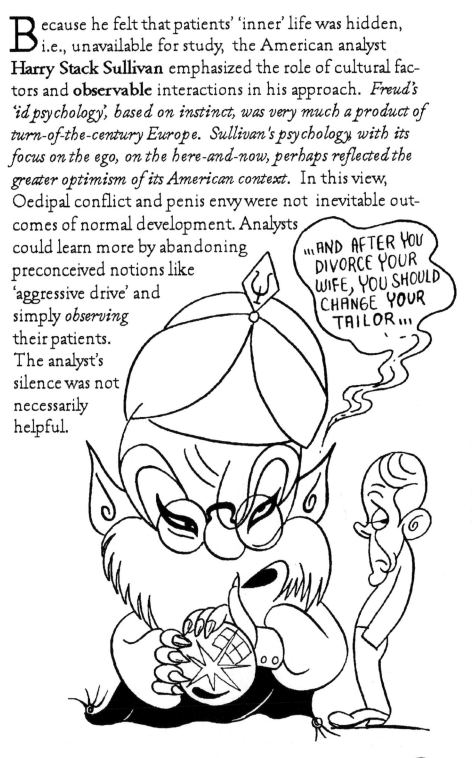

...AND AFTER YOU DIVORCE YOUR WIFE, YOU SHOULD CHANGE YOUR TAILOR...

Erich Fromm felt that the Freudians placed undue emphasis on libido and paid insufficient attention to the individual's relatedness to the world. In *The Sane Society* and *Escape from Freedom* he applied psychoanalytic thinking to urgent social problems.

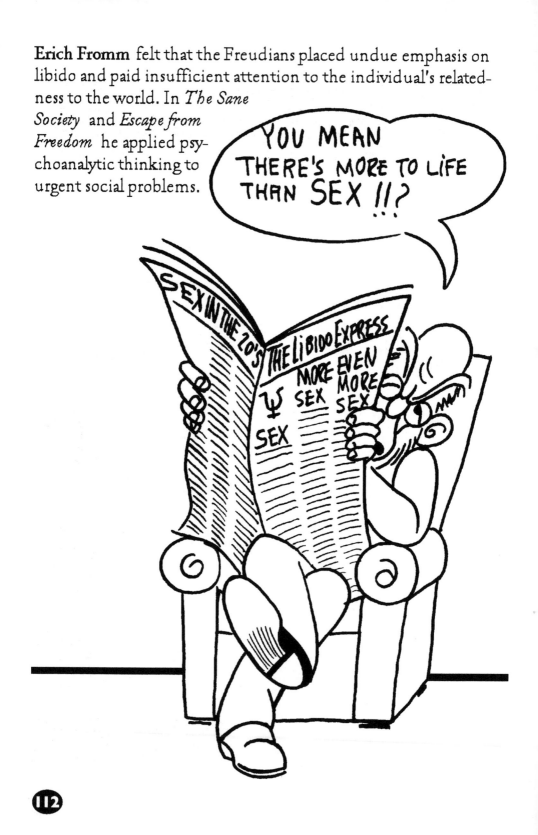

Abraham Maslow believed that man was basically good, and his work focused on 'self-actualization' of the psychiatrically healthy person.

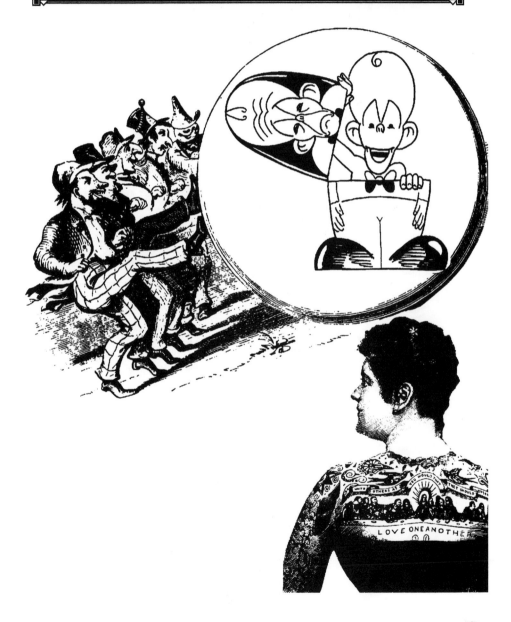

J ean Piaget's work with infants set the stage for a scientific *observational* (instead of merely speculative) approach to childhood development.

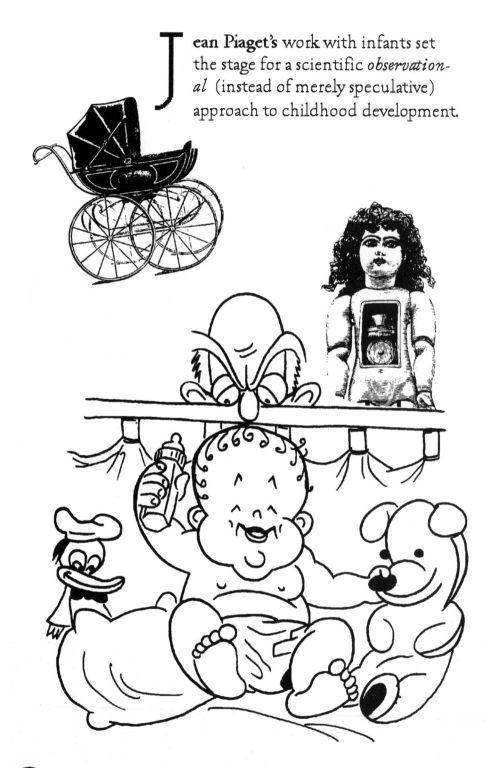

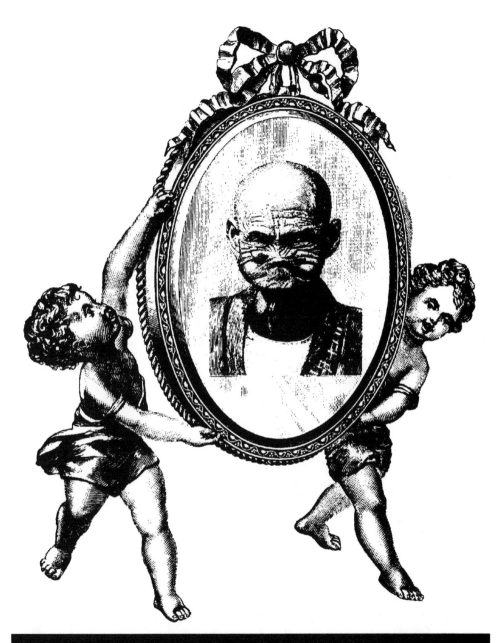

Development continues beyond childhood, throughout the life of the individual, according to ERIK ERIKSON. Erikson described specific 'tasks', such as separation and autonomy, that were appropriate to each developmental stage. His book *Young Man Luther* is a classic of 'psychobiography': life history from a psychoanalytic point of view.

Existential psychiatrists (Victor Frankl and others) align themselves with their patients' search for *meaning*. Choosing an 'authentic' way of life in the face of (a) innumerable doubts and 'existential' anxiety and (b) the certainty of death, is the major task of therapy and of adulthood in general.

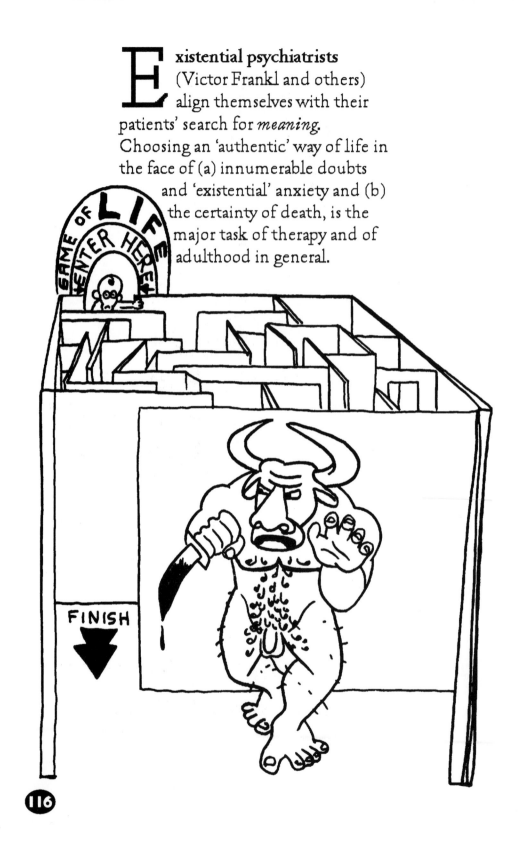

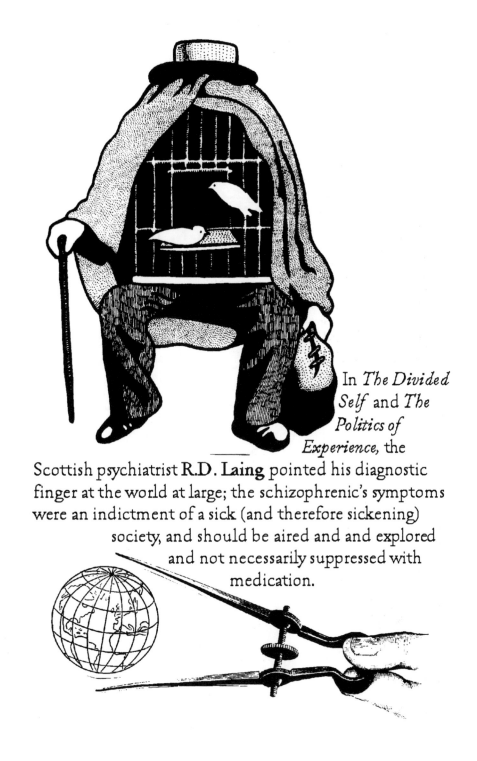

In *The Divided Self* and *The Politics of Experience*, the Scottish psychiatrist **R.D. Laing** pointed his diagnostic finger at the world at large; the schizophrenic's symptoms were an indictment of a sick (and therefore sickening) society, and should be aired and and explored and not necessarily suppressed with medication.

Then there are the 'anti-psychiatrists.' Prominent among them is **Thomas Szasz**, who questions some of the basic assumptions of psychiatry: maybe there is no such thing as mental illness...perhaps psychiatry is nothing more than a sophisticated form of social control!

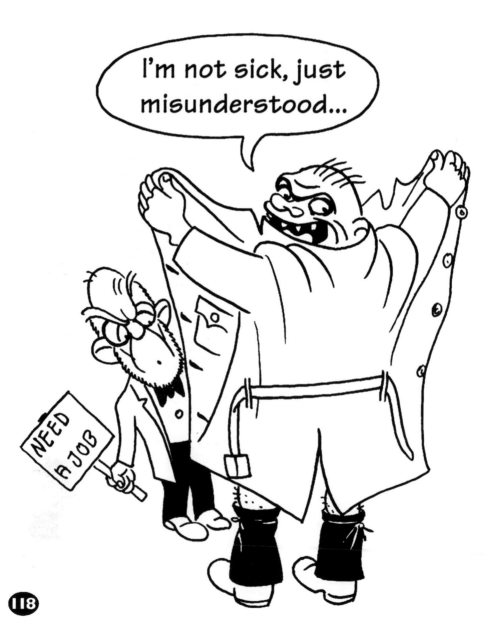

Heinz Kohut, with his emphasis on early (so-called 'pre-Oedipal') problems like separation and attachment has probably done more than anyone else this century to bring psychotherapy back down to earth. According to Kohut, the infant's need for both recognition (*mirroring*) and idealization of the parents can persist throughout life...especially for those with *narcissistic* problems (see below.) In Kohutian 'self psychology' the therapist uses empathy and warmth to treat the patient's fragile self-esteem.

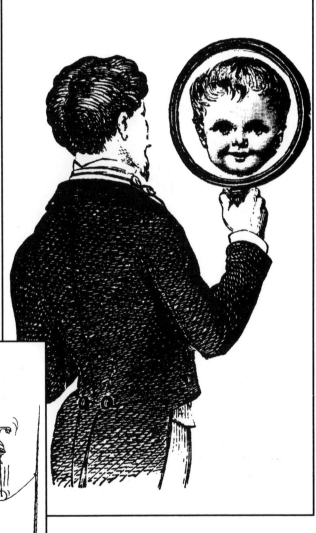

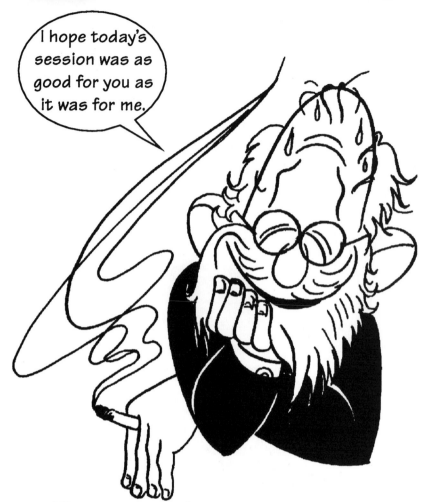

The practitioner of **sex therapy** is often a psychiatrist--though not always.

Problems with sexual performance and intimacy are often highly treatable; sex therapists use a combination of both behavioral and psychotherapeutic techniques.

Group therapy's aim is to change individual behavior by means of *group process.* The idea is that men and women are social animals, embedded in a 'social matrix'; so the most effective way to understand and eventually alter one's behavior is by looking at the kind of interactions we have with others. As with individuals, with time and insight groups evolve, moving from childlike dependence on the leader to autonomy (self-reliance.)

Although group therapies differ widely in structure and approach, usually there is a group leader who facilitates the processes of ventilation, clarification, confrontation, and interpretation. Groups usually have between eight and twelve members, and meet once weekly for one to two hours. The group format has found wide application in the *self-help movement* (Alcoholics Anonymous, Narcotics Anonymous, Overeaters Anonymous, etc.)

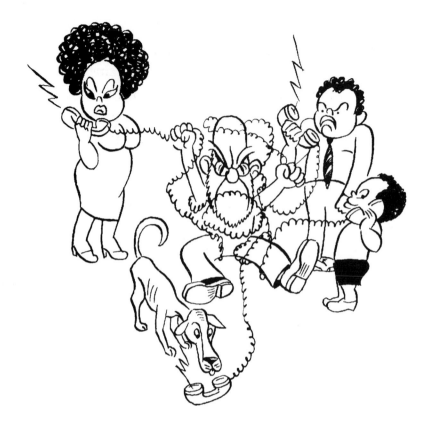

Family therapy looks at and works with the most important influence upon individual development--the family. Like individuals, families function along a spectrum of health and illness. Family therapists attempt to clarify the often confusing messages that family members send one another, and may attempt to reorganize family communications along healthier and more direct lines. Family work is often an integral part of treatment during psychiatric hospitalization.

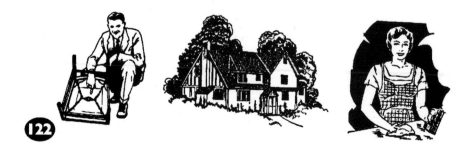

Behavior therapy actually has very little to do with Freud or neo-Freudians. **Ivan Pavlov** demonstrated that a physiological response (the salivation of a dog) could be *conditioned*, i.e. linked, to a formerly neutral stimulus like a ringing bell. Pavlov's successors (**B.F. Skinner** and others) described *operant conditioning* and how it could be used to understand and treat psychiatric disorders.

Motivation and unconscious processes are irrelevant: it's the person's *behavior* that counts. Problems like phobias and compulsions (see below) can be treated by *desensitization* which involves repeated exposure to the anxiety-provoking stimulus until *extinction* (disappearance) of the anxiety response results.

The behaviorist approach has been criticized for its anti-humanist (i.e, man is nothing but a set of behaviors, a black box) slant and for its potential application to totalitarian rule.

B.F.
Skinnner
Fan Club

How about Scientology?
What about EST
(The Forum?)

A number of 'fringe' movements have become popular in recent years, cashing in on the huge numbers of people willing to spend (often exorbitant) amounts of money on their problems. At best, these groups do no harm; at worst, they subject their members to emotional and financial hardship that is anything but therapeutic. An additional danger is that medical problems--which may contribute to or cause emotional ones--go unrecognized, and therefore are untreated.

MENTAL HEALTH
FLEA MARKET

COME ONE
COME ALL

Diagnose

It helps to know as much as possible about the problem that is being treated. That's where *diagnosis* comes in. Of course, this was much less of an issue prior to the 1950's, when available treatments were nonspecific and of unproven benefit.

The history of diagnosing mental disorders is as long and varied as that of psychiatry itself.

Kraepelin's observations on thousands of patients yielded significant information on *course and outcome*. Patients with manic-depressive psychosis were like other patients with manic-depressive psychosis: most could be expected to have illness-free intervals.

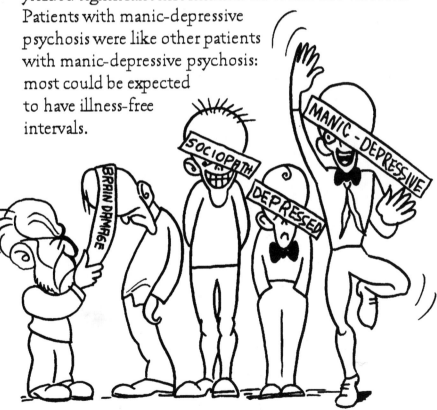

The neurosis vs. psychosis distinction was based on the absence (*neurosis*) or presence (*psychosis*) of delusions or hallucinations, i.e., on the **symptom** picture.

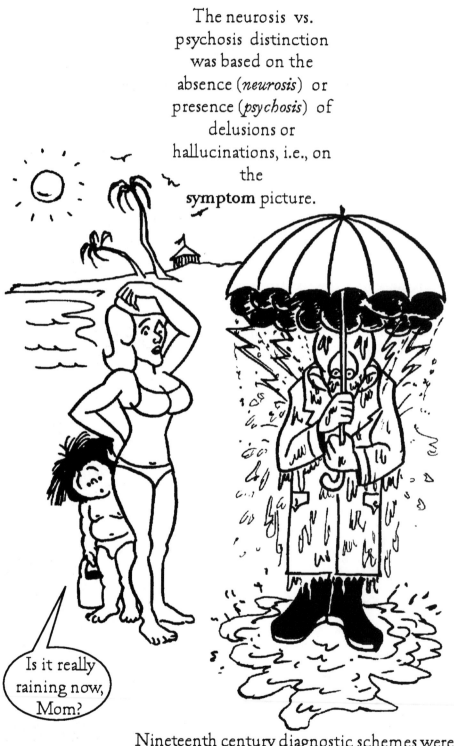

Is it really raining now, Mom?

Nineteenth century diagnostic schemes were elaborate, fanciful and in general not terribly useful.

In the 1950s doctors became more interested in standardizing diagnosis. *The Diagnostic and Statistical Manual (DSM)* was an attempt to do just that. For the first time, psychiatrists from Brazzaville to Brooklyn who used this manual could be reasonably certain that they were talking about the same illnesses.

The original *DSM* (1952) had its problems, and has been revised several times since. (The most recent [1987] edition is *DSM-III-R.*)

DSM is the offspring of a committee of psychiatrists, psychologists and epidemiologists who meet periodically to pool research findings and update clinical observations. The effort is to construct diagnostic categories that are both *valid* (they label what they claim to label) and *reliable* (diagnosis is consistent over time and among patients.) Although not yet universally accepted, *DSM* represents a significant advance over earlier methods based on casual and untested observations.

LET YOUR FINGERS DIAGNOSE...

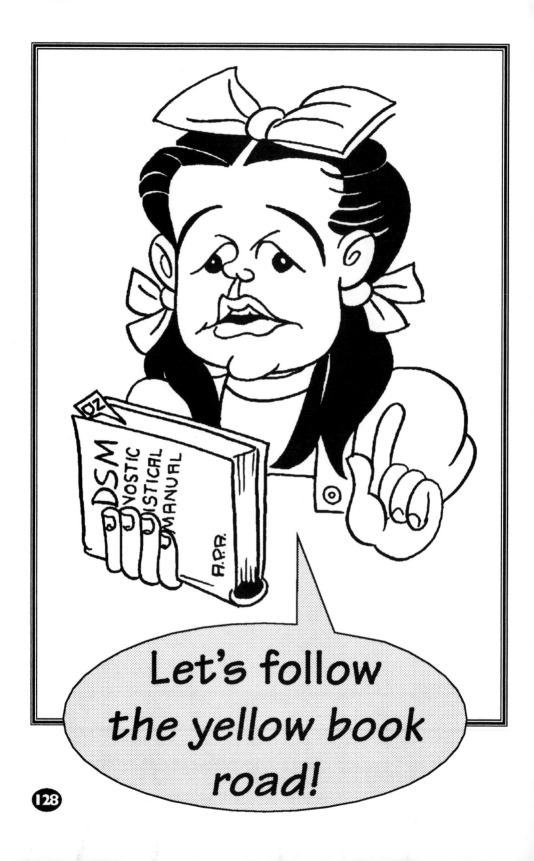

Diagnoses in *DSM-III-R* are organized along 'axes,' which taken together convey more information than a single diagnostic label like 'depression' or 'schizophrenia' ever could.

Axis I lists the major psychiatric disorders, such as depression, mania, schizophrenia, and drug dependence. Patients can have one or more of these at the same time.

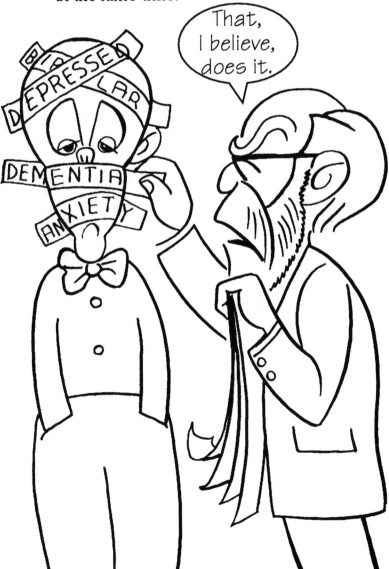

AXIS II:

the personality disorders. Unlike axis I disorders, which can appear suddenly and then remit, personality disorders are 'trait' disorders--characteristic ways of functioning and relating to others that are very resistant to change.

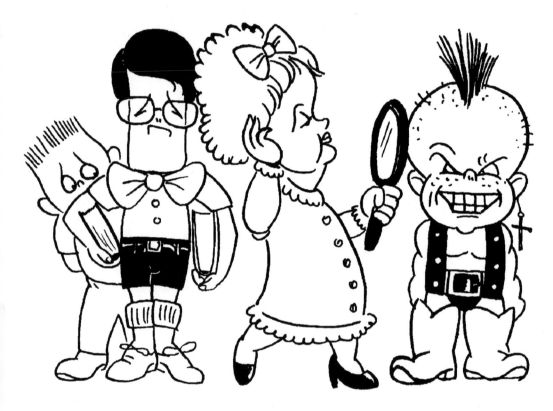

AXIS III:

concurrent physical disorders

AXIS IV:

lists the severity of recent stressors, such as recent job loss or death of a spouse.

AXIS V:
a rating of the individual's overall functioning, on a
scale of 0 (lowest functioning) to 100 (Superman!)

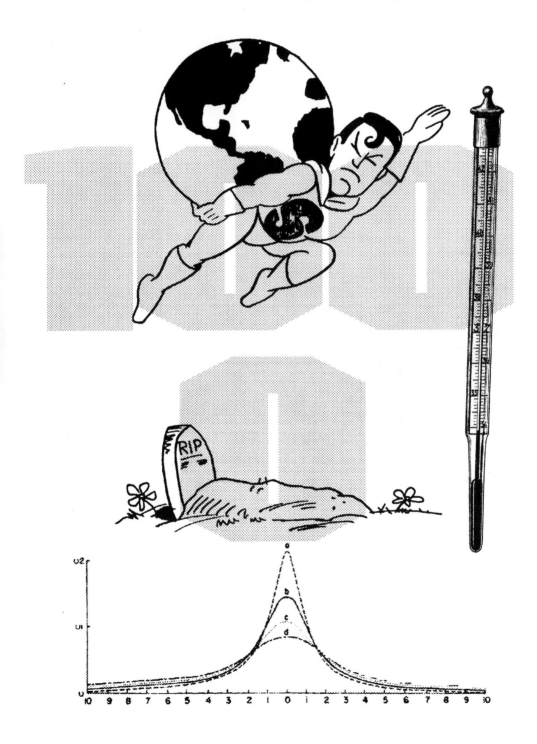

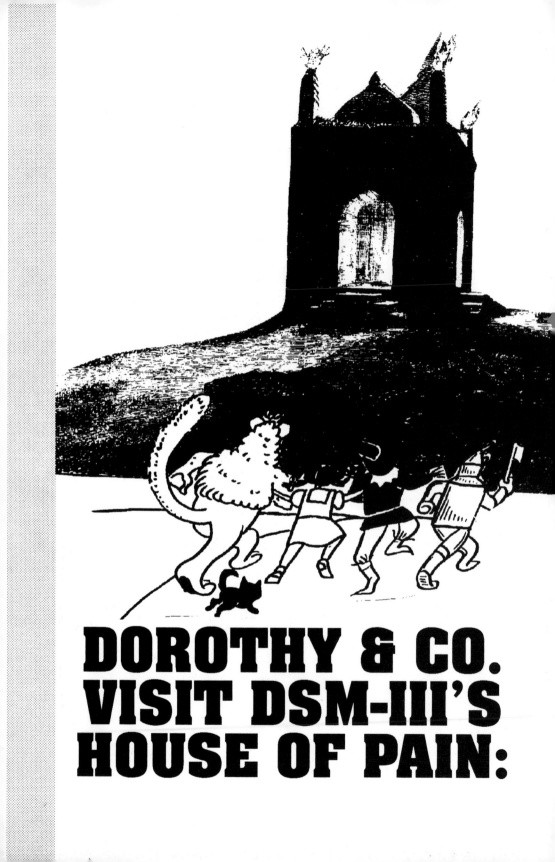

DOROTHY & CO. VISIT DSM-III'S HOUSE OF PAIN:

D epression. Perhaps *the* most common disorder in psychiatry. Different types: 'reactive' (set off by a loss or upset, may clear up when things improve) vs. 'biological' ('endogenous' or 'major' depression.) Symptoms of major depression can include loss of appetite, low energy, insomnia, thoughts of suicide.

DE PRESSION

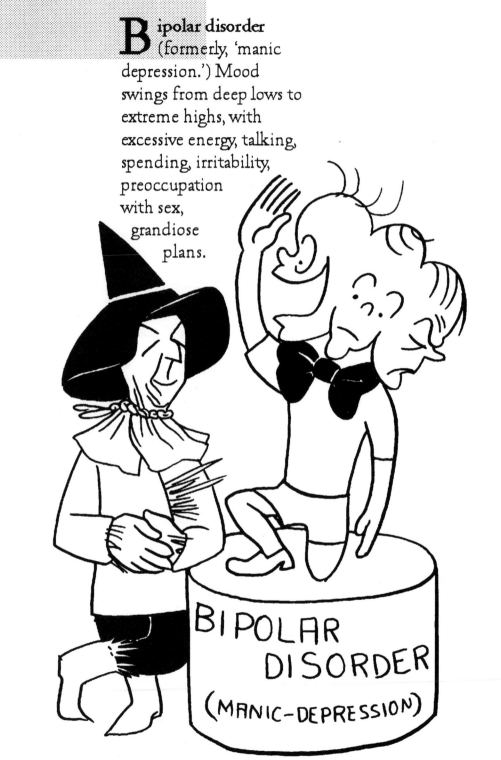

Bipolar disorder (formerly, 'manic depression.') Mood swings from deep lows to extreme highs, with excessive energy, talking, spending, irritability, preoccupation with sex, grandiose plans.

BIPOLAR DISORDER (MANIC-DEPRESSION)

UNIPOLARS only have mood swings in one direction—DOWN!

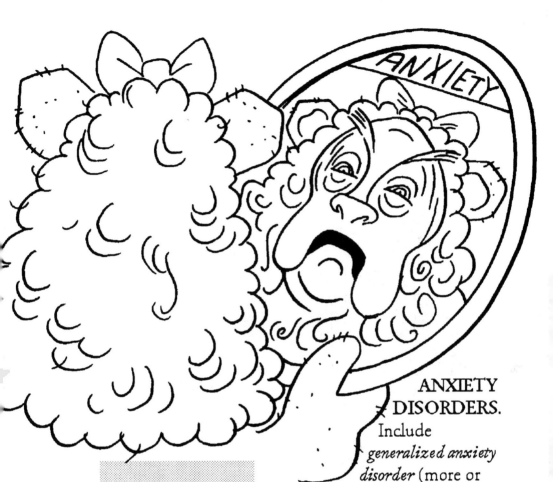

ANXIETY DISORDERS.
Include
generalized anxiety disorder (more or less persistent anxiety states not necessarily related to current stress); *panic disorder* (**panic attacks** = transient episodes of intense fear, sense of impending doom, racing pulse, need to get away); and *obsessive-compulsive disorder* (person experiences extreme anxiety unless he repeats certain behaviors over and over again, such as counting, making lists, or washing hands.)

"You mean, I never really left Kansas?"

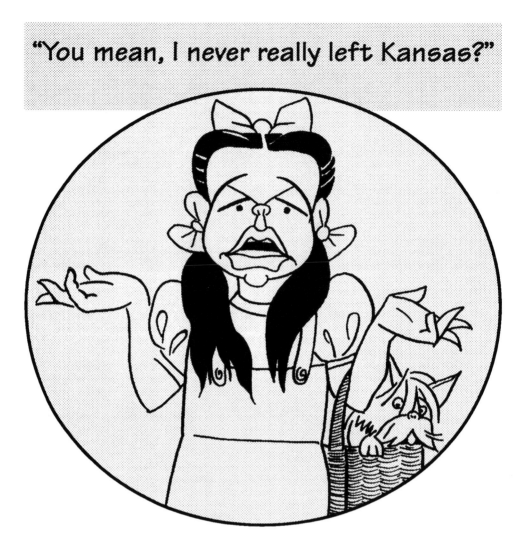

SCHIZOPHRENIA.

Thought disorder (illogical speech,
loosening of associations) and
problems with *reality testing* (persons
sees or hears or believes things that the
rest of us do not.) Often a lifelong
condition with a worsening course.

ORGANIC MENTAL DISORDERS.
(including *delirium* and *dementia* states.)

Problems with speech, behavior and especially memory, due to either temporary or permanent brain damage. Example: *Alzheimer's Disease.*

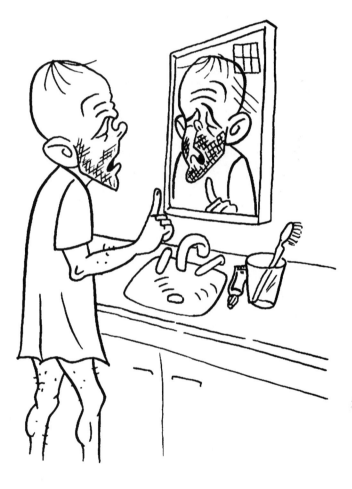

"Have we met before?"

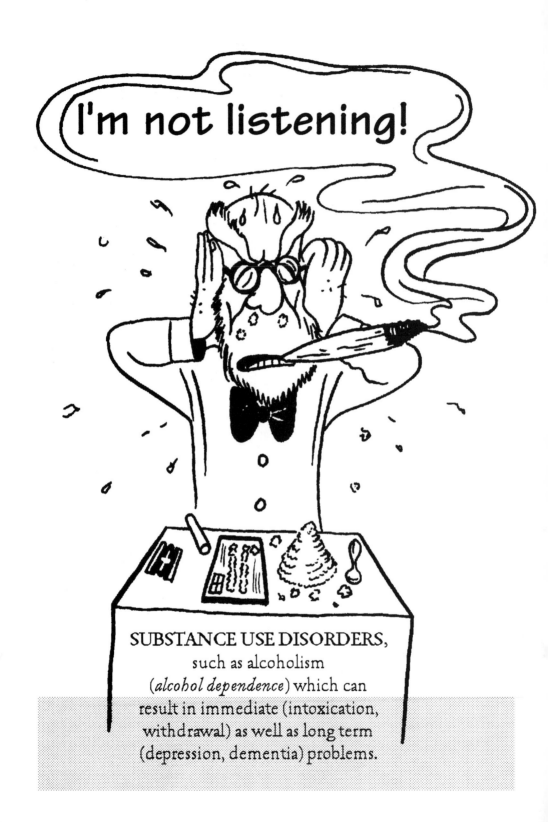

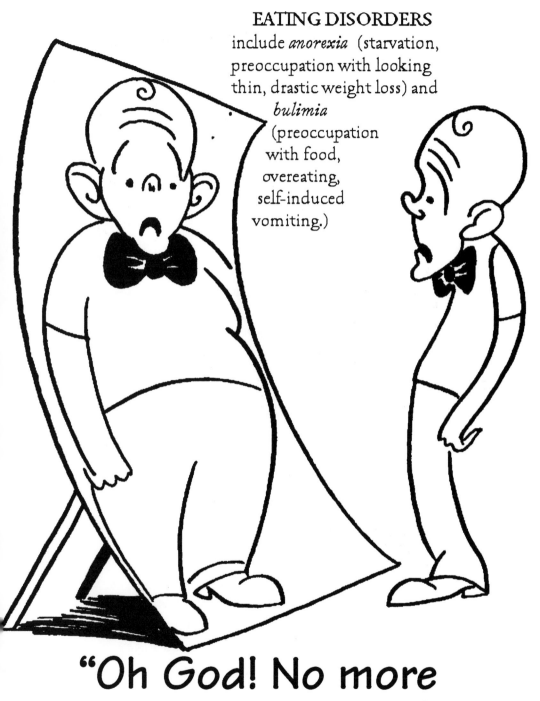

EATING DISORDERS include *anorexia* (starvation, preoccupation with looking thin, drastic weight loss) and *bulimia* (preoccupation with food, overeating, self-induced vomiting.)

"Oh God! No more celery treats for me!"

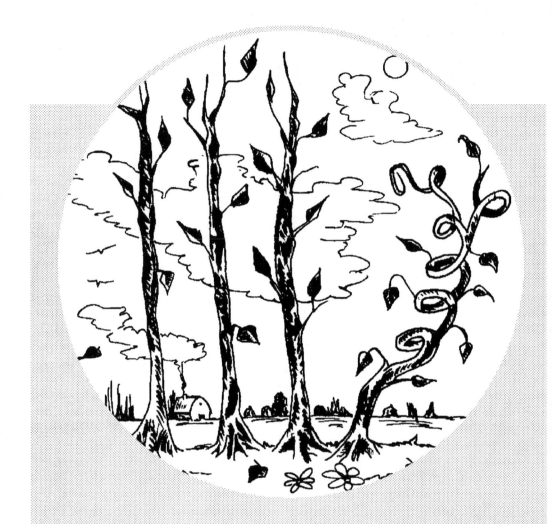

A*ntisocial, histrionic, borderline, narcissistic* and *schizoid* are among the **personality disorders** listed in DSM-III-R. The presence of a personality disorder complicates the evaluation and treatment of other psychiatric problems.

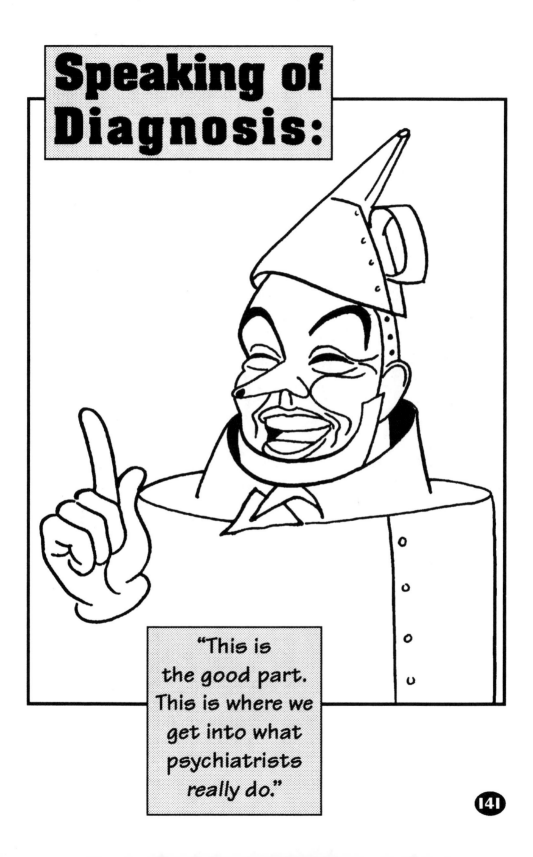

Speaking of Diagnosis:

"This is the good part. This is where we get into what psychiatrists really do."

141

Many medical disorders can either cause or **mimic** psychiatric symptoms. Depression, for example, can be a manifestation of an underlying hormone problem; delirium or dementia can be caused by liver or heart failure. As a physician, the psychiatrist is trained to recognize and treat these situations.

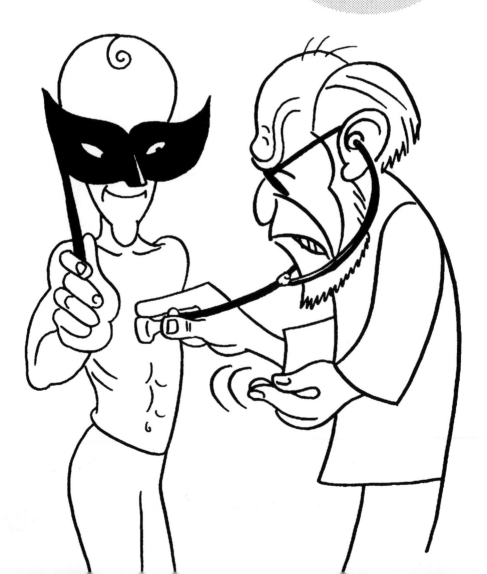

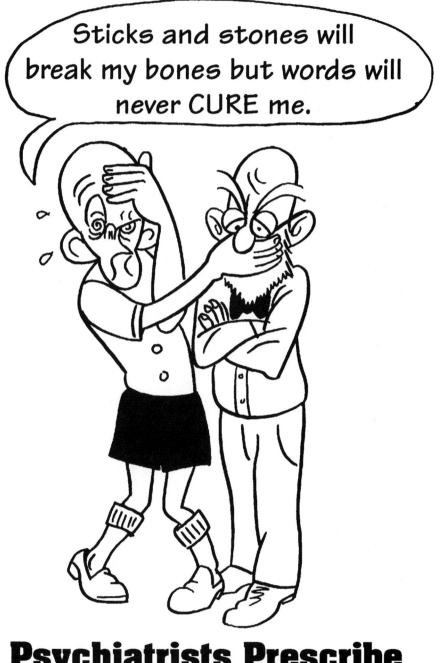

Psychiatrists Prescribe Medication

The introduction of **antidepressant** and **antipsychotic** medication in the 1950's revolutionized the treatment of major mental illness.

Previously, psychiatric interventions for potentially life threatening disorders like depression and schizophrenia had been limited to non-specific sedation and ineffectual talking 'cures.' (While the effectiveness of psychotherapy for less severe conditions remains to be determined, we *do* know that

Just call me Dr. Pill

psychotherapy alone fails miserably with psychoses and severe mood disorders.) For a number of years *insulin shock* (the injection of insulin to produce low blood sugar and seizures) enjoyed a vogue but fortunately this dangerous treatment was eventually abandoned.

In order to better understand how these drugs work, we'll need to take a crash course in

neurochemistry & neurophysiology.

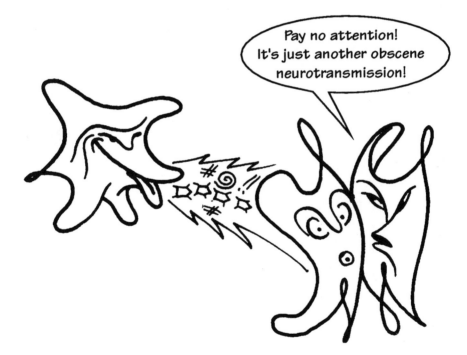

The brain (which at least among psychiatrists is considered the 'master organ' of the body) is not as homogenous as it appears. Under the microscope are revealed literally hundreds of millions of cells, *neurons*, organized into complex pathways that constantly send and receive information.

neurotransmission

The neuron is a link
in a chain of other neurons
(think of it as a microscopic bucket
brigade, with hundreds and sometimes
thousands of connections with other cells.) The
dendrites receive a chemical signal from the *axon*
of the adjacent neuron; this signal is in turn
propagated (transmitted) down the length of the
cell. This results in the release of *neurotransmitter*
molecules from the axon tip across a synaptic space
to the neurotransmitter *receptor* site of the next
neuron, and so on down the line (These events
occur within milliseconds, so that
neurotransmission is very rapid indeed.)

Well, my mother doesn't think so

The neurotransmitters are fairly **simple** molecules; one type of neuron may release only one type of neurotransmitter.

Scientists have been able to identify specific neurotransmitter abnormalities in a number of psychiatric disorders (but these abnormalities are confined to the brain; there is as yet no convenient *blood* test that can identify such problems.)

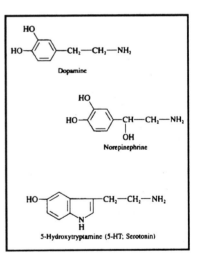

neurotransmitters

Dance of the Neurotransmitters

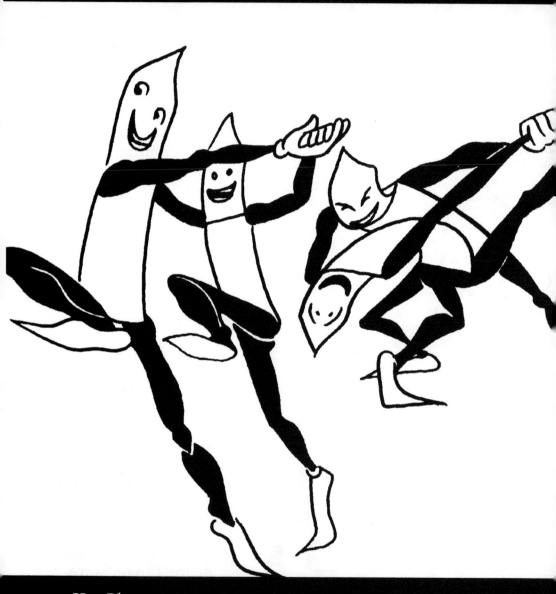

Key Players	Principal Roles
DOPAMINE	activation level, mood, movement
NOREPINEPHRINE	mood, activation level
SEROTONIN	mood, sleep, appetite, aggression
ACETYLCHOLINE	mood (?), autonomic nervous system

...Which takes us right back to the
antipsychotics.

These drugs seem to have a fairly specific effect on psychotic symptoms like hallucinations, delusions and thought disorder. They are also useful in treating severe anxiety and agitation

Bye, I'm out of here, there's no place like home!!

COMMONLY PRESCRIBED ANTIPSYCHOTICS:

*chlorpromazine *perphenazine
*thioridazine *haloperidol
*trifluoperazine
*fluphenazine

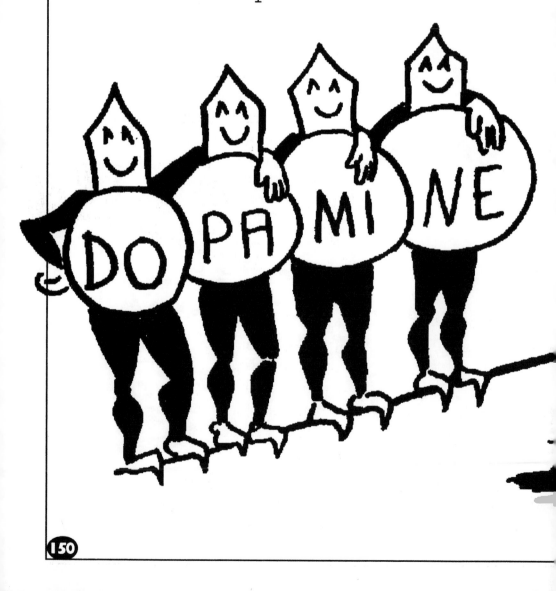

Neuroleptic drugs like *Thorazine, Stelazine,* and *Haldol* are known to block dopamine receptors...which is a good thing, since evidence suggests that there is way too much dopamine activity in psychotic illness. Problem is, dopamine centers in parts of the brain not necessarily related to thinking and thinking problems *are* also affected by these medications. Neuroleptic side effects can include severe muscle spasm, tremor, slowness, and *tardive dyskinesia* (involuntary and sometimes irreversible muscle movements.)

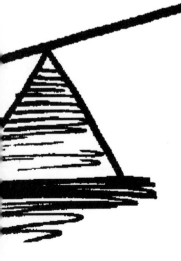

There may be less risk of dyskinesia with *clozapine,* one of the newer antipsychotic medications. Most of these medications are available as injectables, to facilitate use with agitated or noncompliant patients.

Thanks to the **antidepressants** (tricyclics and others), millions of lives have been improved and (literally) saved. These medications, introduced in the late 1950s, seem to work by bolstering levels of neurotransmitters like serotonin and norepinephrine in the brain. Interestingly, the antidepressants take anywhere from one to four weeks to work (the amount of time necessary for brain chemistry changes to occur.) These drugs can be effective not only in depression but in anxiety disorders, panic disorders, and some addictive and eating disorders as well.

The newer antidepressants appear to have fewer side effects than the older, 'first generation' tricyclics.

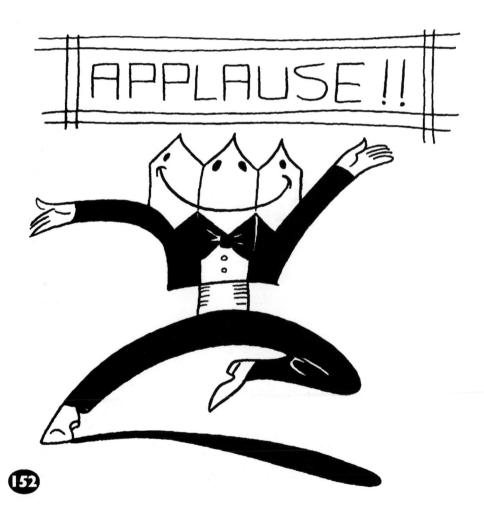

COMMONLY PRESCRIBED ANTIDEPRESENTS:

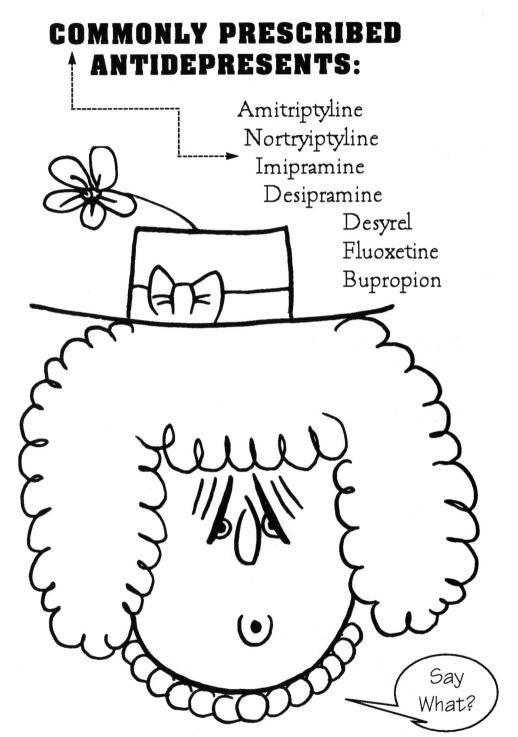

Amitriptyline
Nortryiptyline
Imipramine
Desipramine
Desyrel
Fluoxetine
Bupropion

Say What?

Carbamazepine *(Tegretol)*, an anticonvulsant, is finding wide use in the treatment of both mood disorders and withdrawal states.

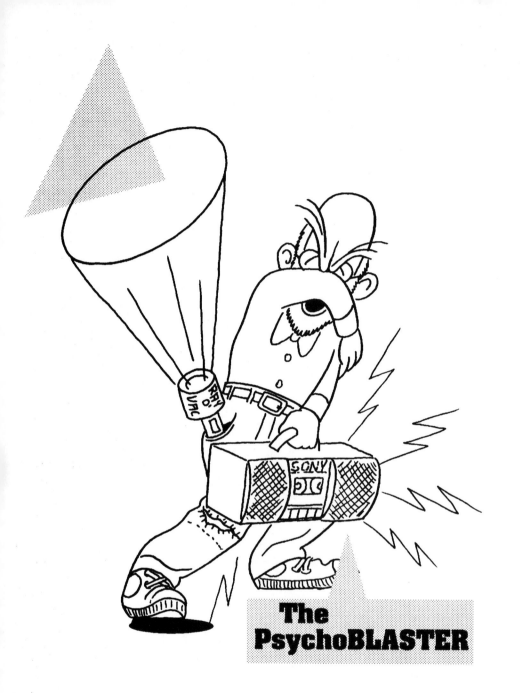

The PsychoBLASTER

Sleep deprivation and phototherapy (bright light therapy)
are used by some psychiatrists to treat mood disorders.

Occasionally patients with severe (life threatening) depressions do not respond to medication. *Electroconvulsive therapy* (ECT), despite its bad reputation, can be a life saving intervention. ECT involves the application of a small amount of electric current to the head, resulting in a 'modified' seizure. Usually six to eight treatments, given two to three times a week, are required. Patients are premedicated so they have no conscious experience of the session and *do not* manifest whole body convulsions.

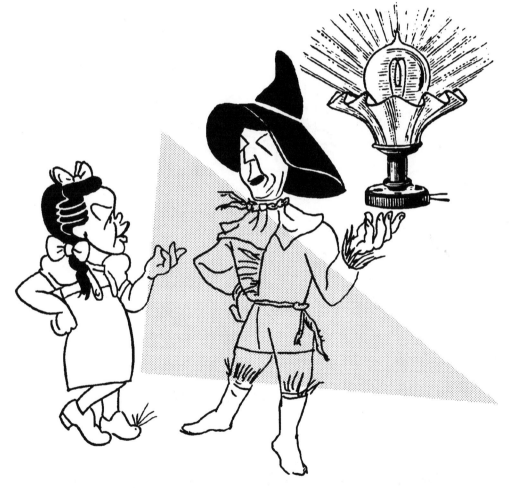

**"Now I'm sorry, but this is absolutely shocking...
You mean ECT is safe?"**

Other Medications

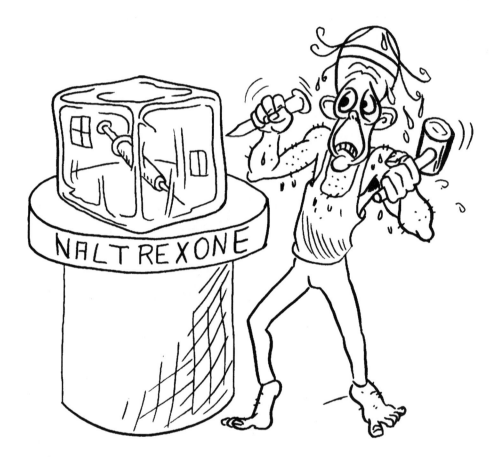

Expanding knowledge of pharmacology and brain receptors has resulted in the development of novel agents--particularly in the treatment of the addictions.

Naltrexone, which acts on brain opiate receptors, literally blocks the heroin high. *Clonidine,* an antihypertensive, has been found to be effective in reducing symptoms of opiate and other types of withdrawal.

Cocainists, who have depleted their neurotransmitters as a result of drug use, may have a more rapid return to health and good functioning with dopamine enhancers like *amantadine*... and certain antidepressants have been found to facilitate recovery not only from major mood disorders but from milder anxiety and depressive states that follow upon cessation of habitual alcohol and drug use.

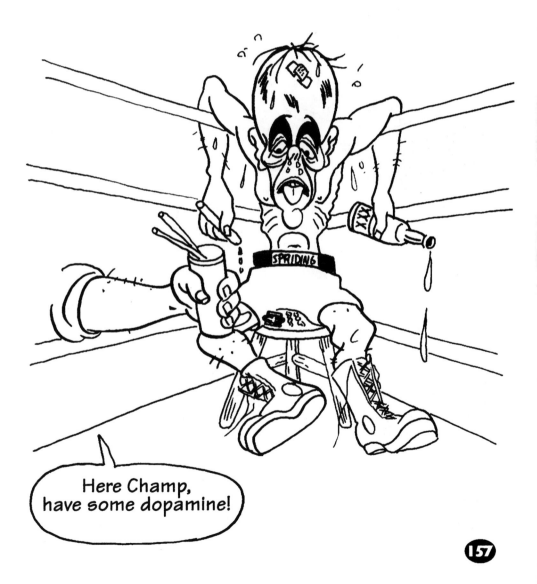

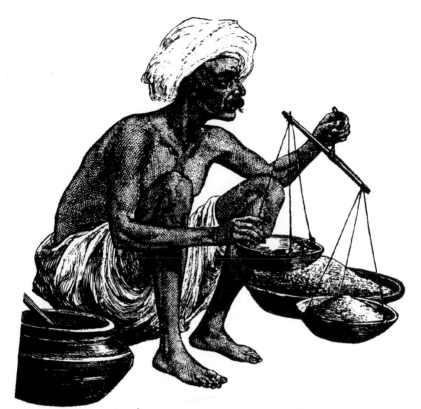

Lithium salts have found great use in the treatment of mood swings (manic-depression, bipolar disorder) and several other conditions; individuals taking lithium must have their blood levels checked periodically.

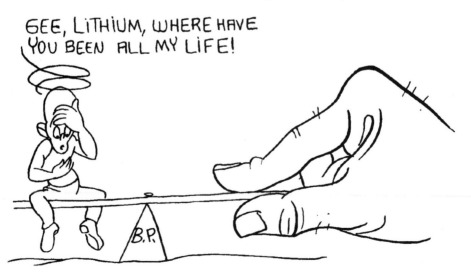

With few exceptions, neither the antipsychotics, the antidepressants nor lithium preparations are habit-forming; there is no danger of physiological **dependence** (tolerance and/or withdrawal.)

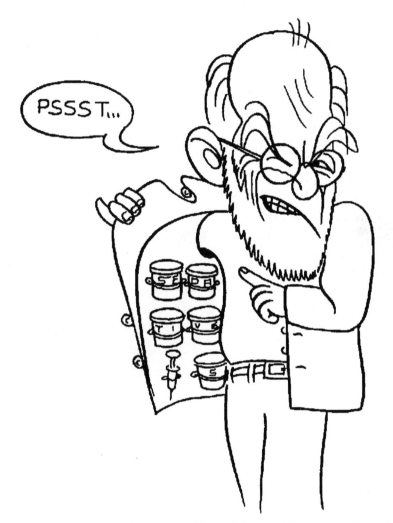

Anti-anxiety medications like Valium (diazepam) and Xanax (alprazolam), members of the *benzodiazepine* class, are likewise very helpful when properly used. Unlike the other drugs discussed above, these are habit-forming and can lead to addictive use. Many psychiatrists give these medications for temporary symptom control, until the co-prescribed antidepressant has a chance to kick in.

Sedative-hypnotics (sleeping pills) include most benzodiazepines, chloral hydrate, and barbiturates like amobarbital and secobarbital. These medications are useful for the short-term (one week or less) treatment of insomnia and have a definite abuse (addictive) potential.

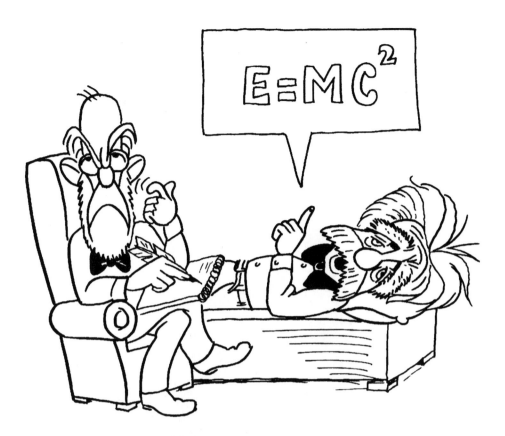

Psychiatric Theory of Relativity

R*elativity* has been a buzzword of the latter part of the twentieth century. Einstein demonstrated how much precise and seemingly 'objective' measurements depended on the observer and upon her point of view.

The same holds true for psychiatry. With increasingly sophisticated epidemiologic and statistical methods, old notions about the 'universality' and prevalence* rates of psychiatric disorders have been overturned.

*Prevalence=how many cases of a particular disease exist in a particular place.

Certain disorders are more common in one part
of the world than another.

Everyone used to think that schizophrenia had
a prevalence of 1%--everywhere in the world.

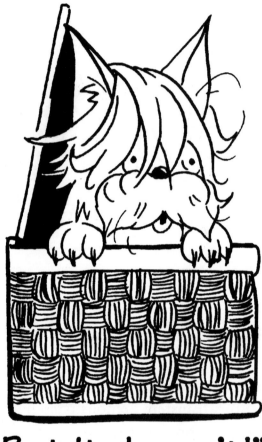

"But it doesn't!"

Example: British psychiatrists tend to diagnose schizophrenia
more often than American psychiatrists.

Diagnostic trends vary even *within* countries. In the U.S.,
doctors question whether certain disorders (i.e., multiple
personality) actually exist, and whether problems like overeating
and destructive use of alchol or drugs should be considered
'legitimate' medical disorders.

"But a disease is a disease is a disease—isn't it? Why all the uncertainty?"

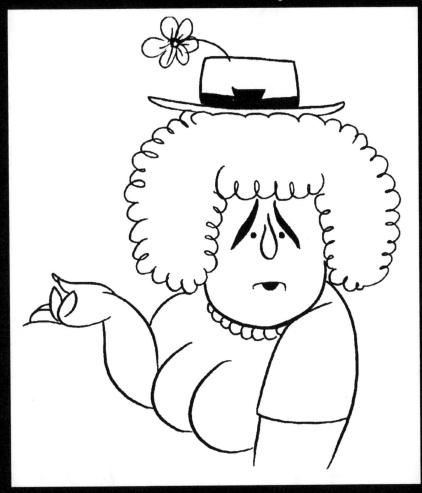

Yes...and no. Although the major psychiatric symptoms are found in all societies, disorders—especially psychiatric ones—are to some extent socially defined.

The psychiatrist, legally empowered to institutionalize individuals against their will, is the gatekeeper of society and its values, of its definitions of 'crazy' and 'sane.'

Researchers still can't agree on how much (if any) influence early childhood experiences have on later development.

And since child rearing practices differ so widely, definitions of 'sickness' and 'health' are going to vary from one culture to the next.

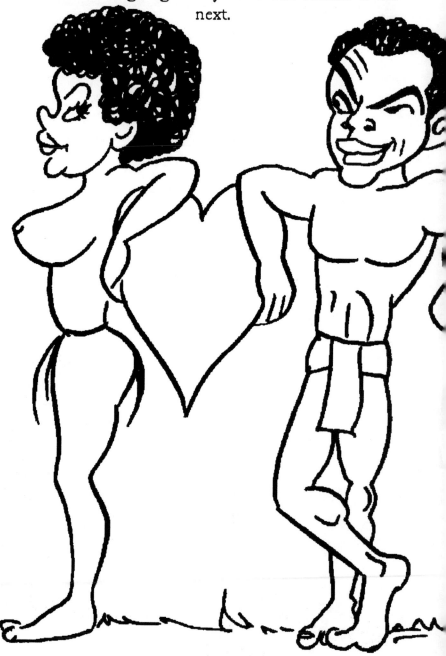

Whatis considered abnormal or deviant in one
culture may not be in another.

Until recently, many Western psychiatrists considered
homosexuality an illness, requiring intensive
psychoanalytic treatment. This attitude would not be
appreciated among the
Sambia of New Guinea,
where male
homosexuality is a
fact of life among
adolescents.

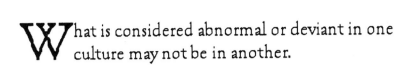

Examples of 'culture-specific' syndromes:

Amok (sudden explosive violence following a period of withdrawal) among Malaysian males...

and *koro* (intense fear among certain Southeast Asian men that their genitals will shrink.)

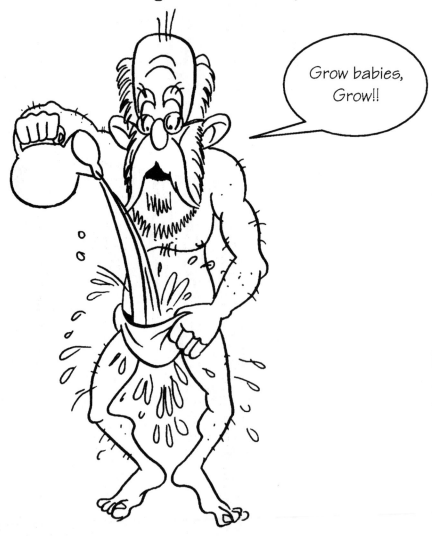

Different cultures favor different ways of expressing pain.

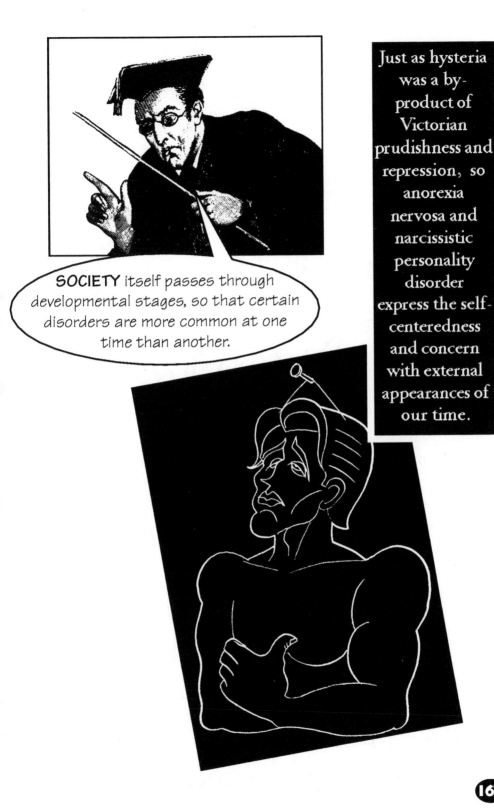

SOCIETY itself passes through developmental stages, so that certain disorders are more common at one time than another.

Just as hysteria was a by-product of Victorian prudishness and repression, so anorexia nervosa and narcissistic personality disorder express the self-centeredness and concern with external appearances of our time.

Diseases are *social* constructions. To a certain but very real extent, patients and patients' 'illness behavior' conform to the expectations of those who treat them. And to complicate matters even further, consider that diagnoses are only *working models,* aimed at achieving the best possible fit between observable symptoms and doctors' theories.

Some feel that the entire framework of Western psychology is outdated--based on old assumptions of male heterosexual superiority--and needs complete revision along feminist or at least egalitarian lines.

HEY, SHUSH MAN!

And as we have seen, theories of illness
change. The diagnostic categories in
DSM-III-R are to a certain extent arbitrary
and will undoubtedly be revised
(and revised and revised.)

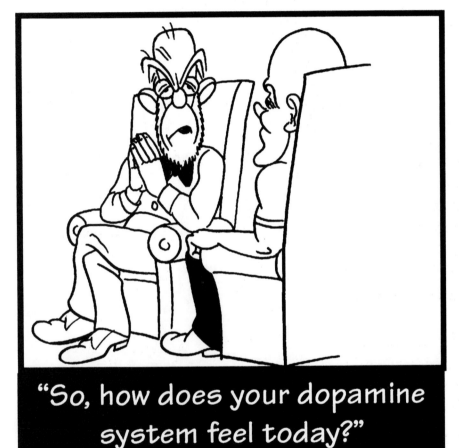

"So, how does your dopamine system feel today?"

Modern science has discarded the medieval humoral theory once
and for all! *Neurotransmitters* are where it's at.

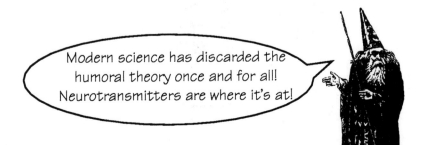

We may never know whether psychiatric disorders are 'caused' by biological factors (such as neurotransmitter problems) or by environmental ones. More than likely, brain chemistry has a powerful effect on behavior--and vice versa. Talking therapies work, and so do medicines. A combination of psychotherapy and medication can be more effective than either intervention alone.

In today's civilized world, psychiatrists have taken on the role of secular 'priests.'

To fulfill this enormous responsibility, psychiatrists must have a healthy respect for the complexity of the psychobiological creature known as man, and never yield to the temptation to endorse a single oversimplified model or approach.

The End

GLOSSARY

abreaction: bringing past emotional conflicts to a head in the present

altruism: helpfulness and charity toward others [a defense mechanism]

anal stage: the first of the four psychosexual growth stages described by Freud. During this period, the infant's main focus is supposedly on defecation and anal sensations

ambivalence: in classical descriptions, a paramount feature of the schizophrenic, who was thought to be unable to choose between alternatives

anthropocentric: attributing human motivations to non-human creatures or events (i.e., an 'angry' hurricane, or an 'altruistic' chimp)

antidepressant: a medication used to treat depression and/or anxiety

antipsychotic: a medication used to treat psychosis

associations: the chain of thoughts and feelings that are associated with a thought or feeling

bipolar disorder: a mood disorder characterized by mood swings in a euphoric and/or irritable and/or depressed direction

castration anxiety: one of the foundations of Freud's theory. Freud believed that little boys feared the loss of the penis; this fear was supposedly provoked by the sight of the female genitals, which were perceived as a lack or loss of male genitals

catharsis: an emotional unburdening, such as takes place when a therapist's skillful interpretation results in the expression of pent up thoughts and feelings

conditioning: originally described by Pavlov, who conditioned dogs to salivate at the sound of a bell by means of the simultaneous presentation of food

death instinct: *thanatos*, an urge toward self-destruction, thought by Freud in his later years to exist side-by-side with *libido*, or life instinct

defense mechanism: a strategy used to keep painful thoughts and feelings out of awareness

dementia praecox: the original term for schizophrenia, which was said to lead to a premature loss of intellectual faculties

denial: disavowal to self or others of some fundamental aspect of thought or behavior ("I don't have a problem with drugs. My wife and doctor and police officer do.") Another of the defense mechanisms.

depression: a loss of appetite for life, ranging from mild ('Sometimes I feel blue') to life threatening ('I'm going to kill myself.')

diagnosis: the label given by a physician to explain a set of problems or abnormal findings in a patient

drive: a pressure that is fundamental to survival of the individual or the species, such as aggression, or sex

ego: a hypothetical agency of the mind which functions to execute the drives

fixation: failure to develop beyond (getting stuck at) any of the earlier psychosexual stages

forensic: legally oriented (forensic psychiatrists work with incarcerated patients)

genital stage: the last of the four psychosexual growth stages described by Freud. During this period, the individual supposedly comes to terms with the more immature longings (i.e., oral, anal, and phallic) and is able to enjoy full 'genital' (=mature) sexuality

hypochondriasis: persistent or repeated physical complaints in the absence of demonstrable physical illness

hysteria: persistent or repeated neurologic complaints (such as weakness or numbness) in the absence of demonstrable neurologic illness.

id: a hypothetical agency of the mind which houses the libidinal and aggressive drives

libido: usually thought of as sex drive, but more inclusively considered as appetite (for life, for sex, for aggression, etc.)

mania: episodes of expansive or irritable or euphoric mood which persist and which can involve diminished need for sleep, increased spending and interest in sex, and grandiose ideas

manic depression: repeated mood swings in the depressed or manic direction (now considered a variant of bipolar disorder)

mind: [your guess is as good as ours!]

narcissism: a persistent set of beliefs in which others are seen as mere extensions of the self; narcissistic individuals have little empathy for others and consequently are lonely and liable to extremes of self-aggrandizement and self-deprecation. Now considered to be a personality disorder.

nervous breakdown: a vague phrase, which could mean an episode of depression or psychosis or many other things besides

neuroleptic: an antipsychotic medication

neurosis: an old term for mental symptoms resulting from inadequately resolved conflicts

oedipus complex: according to Freud, a normal part of every boy's development, featuring the boy's wish to have sex with his mother and to murder his father

oral stage: the second of Freud's psychosexual growth stages, in which the baby's libido is primarily focused on the mouth and on its functions (eating, sucking, drinking)

organic mental disorder: a mental disorder, such as Alzheimer's disease, or alcoholic dementia, in which there is demonstrable damage to or alteration of the brain

paraphilia: perversion

parapraxis: an unintended behavior (such as leaving one's keys somewhere, or a slip of the tongue) considered to have an unconscious motivation

pathology: deviation from the norm

personality disorder: a relatively enduring set of traits, such as obsessionality, or preoccupation with the self, which comes to psychiatric attention. These are operationally defined in the *DSM-III-R* diagnostic manual

phallic stage: the second of the psychosexual growth stages described by Freud, characterized by a behavioral emphasis on phallic (=penis, or penis-like) behavior such as poking or prodding

preconscious: in Freud's earlier topographic model of the mind, the area containing thoughts and feelings just below the level of conscious awareness

projection: attributing thoughts and feelings of one's own to others [a defense mechanism]

psychoanalysis: a regular and usually frequent series of meetings between patient and analyst in which the latter analyses the unconscious motivations of the former's thoughts, feelings, dreams, and behavior

psychopharmacology: the study and application of drugs which affect mood and intellect and behavior

psychosis: a deficit in reality testing, or departure from commonly held beliefs about and perceptions of the world (i.e., delusions, hallucinations)

rationalization: an (often) elaborate justification of an emotionally or unconsciously motivated act [a defense mechanism]

repetition compulsion: considered a primary feature of neurosis, this is described as a need to repeat, in the here-and-now, unresolved situations and conflicts from the past

repression: suppression, to the point of forgetting, of some fact or experience or subjective state [a defense mechanism]

structural model: Freud's later model of the mind, featuring the components *id, ego,* and *superego*; this replaced his previous topographic model

sublimation: the substitution of a more socially sanctioned activity (such as painting) for a more 'primitive' one (such as smearing feces)

superego: that agency of the mind posited by Freud as the 'watchdog' or conscience, either rewarding individuals for their behavior with self-approbation, or punishing them with guilt

thanatos: see Death Instinct

transference: the set of feelings that usually evolve on the part of the patient toward the therapist, which often provide a focus for the work of therapy

tricyclic: a type of antidepressant medication, so-called because of the chemical structure which includes three benzene rings linked side-to-side

unconscious: the mind's repository of each day's accumulation of longings, perceptions, feelings, and thoughts; the sphere of mental activity next to or beneath that of ordinary waking consciousness

unipolar disorder: episodes of mood swings that occur in only one direction (usually depression)

REFERENCES

Ackerknecht, Erwin Heinz. *A Short History of Psychiatry* (translated by Sula Wolff.) New York, Hafner Publishing Co., 1968

Breggin, Peter R. *Toxic Psychiatry.* New York, St. Martin's Press, 1991.

Brenner, Charles. *An Elementary Textbook of Psychoanalysis* (rev. ed.) Garden City, Anchor Press, 1974.

Erikson, Erik H. *Childhood and Society* (Second edition.) New York, Norton, 1963.

Frank, Jerome. *Persuasion and Healing: A Comparative Study of Psychotherapy.* Baltimore, The Johns Hopkins University Press, 1973

Freud, Anna. *The Ego and the Mechanisms of Defense* (Revised edition.) New York, International Universities Press, 1966.

Freud, Sigmund. *The Interpretation of Dreams* (translated by A.A.. Brill.) New York, Modern Library, 1950.

Jung, C.G. *Modern Man in Search of a Soul.* New York, Harcourt, Brace & World, 1934.

Kaplan, Harold I, Sadock Benjamin J. *Comprehensive Textbook of Psychiatry* (5th ed.) Baltimore, Williams & Wilkins, 1989.

Kohut, Heinz. *The Analysis of the Self.* New York, International Universities Press, 1966.

Laing, R.D. *The Divided Self: A Study of Sanity and Madness.* Chicago, Quadrangle Books, 1960.

Minuchin, Salvador. *Families & Family Therapy.* Cambridge, Mass., Harvard University Press, 1974.
Szasz, Thomas S. *The Myth of Mental Illness: Foundations of a Theory of Personal Conduct.* New York, Hoeber-Hoeber, 1961.

Tarachow, Sidney. *An Introduction to Psychotherapy.* International Universities Press, Madison, 1963.

Yalom, Irvin D. *The Theory and Practice of Group Psychotherapy* (2nd ed.) Basic Books, New York, 1975

Zilboorg, Gregory, George Henry. *A History of Medical Psychology.* New York, W.W. Norton & Co., 1941

INDEX